BALANCED LIFE

FOR PROPER AND EFFECTIVE WEIGHT MANAGEMENT

BY

INNOCENT KARIKOGA

BALANCED LIFE

2

Published by

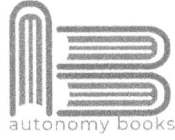

autonomy books

in collaboration with

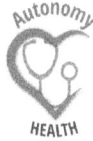

Autonomy
HEALTH

No part of this publication may be reproduced, stored in a retrieval system, or transmitted in any form or by any means, electronic, mechanical, photocopying, and recording or otherwise, without the prior written permission of the author, except for brief passages in connection with a review written for publication or inclusion in a print or online medium, magazine, newspaper, periodical, or broadcast. To perform any of the aforementioned is an infringement of copyright law.

This publication provides content related to educational, medical, and psychological topics; however, it is not intended to substitute for the medical advice of a licensed physician. The reader should consult with their physician on any health-related matters. All health-related issues require medical supervision. It is the reader's responsibility to comply with current and future medical treatments and advice.

Further, understand that the guidance contained herein is not intended as a substitute for consultation with a licensed medical, educational, or health care professional. Using the material implies the acceptance of this disclaimer. Before beginning any change in lifestyle in any way, it is recommended to consult a licensed professional to ensure that you are doing what is best for your health.

This book intends to enlighten readers with a simplified, basic understanding of weight management and how weight generally affects our bodies.

The information found in this book is refined excerpts from the most recent editions of some of the most comprehensive medical textbooks. No claims without scientific basis are found in this book.

Revised edition.

ISBN: 978-1-0689798-6-6

1. Introduction

Gone are the days when having a belly that jiggled like a bowl of royal jelly wasn't just acceptable—it was desirable. Back then, being overweight wasn't a cry for help or a side effect of binge-watching your favourite TV show with a bag of chips. No, it was a flex. A sign that you had enough wealth to feast while everyone else gnawed on tree bark and dreams.

For most of history, however, the average Joe and Jane weren't rolling in surplus calories. They were too busy rolling stones to build pyramids or chasing after squirrels with sticks to worry about whether their BMI fell in the "ideal" range. These folks lived in perpetual cardio mode—hunting, gathering, and desperately hoping their next meal didn't scamper away or fight back.

Refrigerators weren't even a twinkle in humanity's eye. If they did manage to catch something edible, it had to be eaten fast—before it spoiled, got stolen, or was "generously" shared with the village. The invention of agriculture gave a glimmer of hope. Now, humans could grow food instead of constantly playing "catch me if you can" with dinner. But Mother Nature, ever the diva, made sure agriculture came with strings attached: pests, droughts, and, of course, seasons.

Seasons meant that sometimes you had an abundance of food, and other times, well...you got to enjoy the culinary adventure of "air pie" and "imagination stew." Hunger and malnutrition were less of a rare tragedy and more of a recurring guest star in the sitcom of survival.

So, while our ancestors might have dreamed of chubbiness as a status symbol, most were stuck being lean—not because they wanted to rock abs but because their lifestyles didn't allow for snack breaks. And now here we are, in the age of all-you-can-eat buffets, glorifying intermittent fasting like it's some new revolutionary idea. History, you cruel jokester.

Hunting and gathering food weren't just a lifestyle—they were a full-time job with terrible benefits. Chasing meat involved hours of stalking, running, and the occasional realization that you were now the prey. Even if you managed to bring home the prehistoric bacon, you still had to devour it because refrigeration wasn't exactly a Stone Age invention. Add to that the competition from your neighbour—who also had a spear and no chill—and meat was more of a seasonal treat than a daily indulgence.

Crops, on the other hand, were the dependable, slightly boring partner in humanity's relationship with food. Plant a seed, wait a bit (provided Mother Nature wasn't in one of her hurricane-mood-swings), and voilà—dinner! Sure, crops weren't as exciting as a freshly roasted mammoth steak, but they didn't try to run away or gore you during harvest season. Plus, they were the ultimate team players in a reliable, albeit carb-heavy, diet.

Now, toss in back-breaking work, laughable wages, and a diet heavy on grains and veggies with only fleeting appearances from meat, and voilà: your average ancient person was rocking the kind of physique modern gym-goers dream of, whether they liked it or not. Fast forward to the 21st century, and the tables have turned. Today, the Western world has made being overweight as common as overpriced lattes and TikTok trends.

But here's the kicker: whether you were a wealthy lord feasting on roast boar or a modern human juggling meal prep with Uber Eats, being overweight has always been the body's way of saying, *"Hey, we need to talk."* It's not great for your joints, heart, or existential dread. Whether it's ancient famine or modern fast food, the message has always been clear: balance is key—assuming, of course, you can still balance.

Once the domain of health professionals armed with scientific facts and helpful advice, body weight is now a social minefield where everyone is an expert, and nobody agrees. Forget BMI charts or dietary guidelines—modern weight discourse has less to do with calories and more about who's "winning" the social commentary Olympics.

In theory, weight is a neutral concept rooted in biology: **calories in, calories out, rinse and repeat.** But in practice, it's become a battleground of societal expectations, personal insecurities, and enough unsolicited opinions to crash a Twitter server. It's no longer just about health; it's about navigating a minefield of social implications that can trigger physical, physiological, and psychological stress faster than you can say, *"Are you really going to eat that?"*

What started as a noble mission to promote public health has somehow morphed into a blunt instrument of social destruction. Discussing weight has gone from a scientific conversation to a game of linguistic gymnastics, where you try to address a critical issue without offending anyone or setting off a Twitter storm.

Let's face it: cramming all the scientific, social, and emotional baggage of weight into one conversation is like trying to carry all your groceries in one trip—overambitious and likely to end in disaster. But if weight has such profound implications for health and society, shouldn't we figure out a way to talk about it that doesn't make everyone feel like they've just lost a round of emotional dodgeball?

The goal should be an inclusive conversation in which facts aren't weapons and everyone feels like they can pull up a chair without judgment. At the end of the day, we're all just trying to carry our own weight—literally and figuratively—without breaking under the pressure.

Once upon a time, someone had a brilliant idea: let's find the most "aesthetically pleasing" woman in the land, crown her with enough rhinestones to blind a small country, and send her off to save the world. What could possibly go wrong? The beauty pageants were meant to be fun, a lighthearted affair with smiling faces, spangled gowns, and the occasional dramatic wave. The winner, armed with her sash and a vague title of "goodwill ambassador," would then embark on a mission to champion social causes.

But here's the kicker: intentions and consequences rarely RSVP to the same party. Instead of fostering goodwill, these beauty pageants unwittingly sent a subtle, insidious message: *This is what beauty looks like. If you don't look like this, better luck next year.*

Suddenly, the rhinestone-studded winner wasn't just a goodwill ambassador—she became the unofficial yardstick of beauty. And while no pageant judge explicitly handed out a "You're Not Beautiful" participation ribbon, the indirect message was hard to miss. For those with a different body type or size, the mirror started to look less like a reflection and more like a funhouse distortion.

Some folks argue that anyone upset by these events should just "get over it." Sure, if only human insecurities could be shrugged off like a bad haircut. But when the same message is served up on repeat—on stage, in magazines, on billboards—it's hard not to feel like it's personally addressed to you, signed "Society."

The real tragedy is that these unintended consequences didn't just derail body positivity; they killed any hope of a civilized conversation about obesity. Weight, once a matter of health and sociology, became a beauty pageant subplot. Now, any attempt to discuss weight is overshadowed by debates about beauty standards, leaving us stuck in a never-ending cycle of tiaras and misunderstandings.

So here we are, trying to address critical social issues while drowning in a sea of glitter and misplaced priorities. Maybe it's time to retire the crowns and focus on the causes they were supposed to represent—without the unspoken message that beauty is a one-size-fits-all affair.

For decades, healthcare professionals have been shouting from the rooftops (and examination rooms) about the adverse health effects of being overweight. Armed with charts, studies, and enough medical jargon to give a dictionary a nervous breakdown, they've tried to keep the conversation grounded in science.

But here's the rub: whenever the word **obesity** enters the conversation, people tend to veer off course faster than a GPS with a low battery. Instead of focusing on the scientific and medical implications, the discussion often swerves into the perilous territory of social connotations. Suddenly, what was meant to be a conversation about health metrics became a minefield of opinions, judgments, and societal baggage.

It's not that people are wrong to feel the weight (pun intended) of the word's social implications. Words carry meaning, after all, and obesity has been weaponized in ways that make it feel more like a judgment than a diagnosis. But in the rush to debate its cultural context, we risk losing sight of its original purpose: to describe a medical condition with measurable health consequences.

Think of it like this: if a doctor warns you about high cholesterol, you're not likely to interpret it as a comment on your social status or self-worth. Yet, obesity carries an emotional charge that turns what should be a straightforward health conversation into a complicated dance of defensiveness and deflection.

Sure, we can't ignore the social layers, but let's not allow them to drown out the science. Obesity isn't a personality flaw, a moral failing, or a character judgment—it's a medical condition with real-world consequences. And while the word might make some people bristle, the stakes are too high to let discomfort dictate the dialogue.

So, the next time obesity comes up, maybe we can agree to keep one foot in the science and the other on the unsteady ground of social perception. Balance might be tricky, but it's better than tripping over our own assumptions.

Body Mass Index (BMI) is the universal scorecard for your body's feud between height and weight. BMI is your weight in kilograms divided by the square of your height in meters. It's simple math, unless you're bad at math, in which case, there's an app for that.

For decades, researchers have agreed that a BMI between **18 and 25** is the sweet spot for optimum health. It's the VIP lounge of body ratios, associated with **fewer cancers**, **heart problems**, **strokes**, and even the dreaded **type 2 diabetes mellitus** (T2DM). Think of it as your body's "Goldilocks Zone"—not too heavy, not too light, just right. But step outside that range, and the plot thickens. Literally.

A BMI **below 18** is a red flag for being **underweight**. Sure, it sounds like a compliment in certain circles, but it's a ticket to a lifetime of **increased disease risk** and **reduced life expectancy**. "Skinny Legend" loses its charm when paired with a vitamin deficiency.

Between 25 and 30? Welcome to the "**Overweight** Zone," where risks for heart disease, strokes, and autoimmune disorders start creeping up like unwanted party guests. Still, you're not in the danger zone yet—you've just ordered appetizers at the buffet of bad health outcomes.

Now, cross into **BMI 30+,** and things get real. This is where obesity makes its dramatic entrance, complete with increased risks of every terrifying disease your doctor can name. And if your BMI hits **40+**, congratulations—you've unlocked **morbid obesity**. It's the final boss of body fat, where even your life expectancy starts waving a white flag.

Here's another kicker: you can't do anything about your height once puberty packs up and leaves. Your weight, though? That's a wildcard, capable of sending your BMI on a rollercoaster ride that could rival the stock market.

So, while BMI is a handy tool, it's not the whole story of your health. But if yours is creeping toward morbid obesity territory, maybe it's time to rethink that second donut. Or third. Or...you get the idea.

Sure, everyone loves to talk about the fat they can see—the muffin tops, double chins, and the spare tires. But the real sneaky villain? The fat inside your blood. This internal saboteur doesn't care how many layers of Spanx you own; it's too busy clogging up your arteries and throwing cholesterol parties in your bloodstream.

Now, there's a well-documented connection between BMI over 25 and bad cholesterol. For those keeping score, about 80% of people with T2DM are at least overweight. It's a straightforward narrative: bigger waistlines equal bigger problems. But let's pause for a reality check, shall we?

If 80% of T2DM patients are overweight, that leaves us with 20% who are either healthy weight or underweight. Yep, a solid chunk of people with T2DM defy the stereotype. It's like discovering that 20% of men don't like sex—it's unexpected and worth looking into.

So, what's going on with that 20%? Could T2DM be about more than just weight? (Spoiler: it is.) While it's easy to laser-focus on the 80%—because who doesn't love dealing with the majority? — it's inherently lazy to dismiss the minority. Ignoring the lean diabetics is like blaming a leaky roof on the rain, saying, *"If it rains enough, some of it is bound to crip into the house."*

Diseases like T2DM aren't just about numbers on a scale or tape measure. They're deeply rooted in the chaos happening inside your blood vessels. Sure, excess weight is a major factor—it's like giving your body's metabolic system a malfunctioning alarm clock. However, weight alone isn't the sole culprit, and relying on correlation as proof of causation is a rookie mistake.

So, the next time someone tells you T2DM is a "fat person's disease," remind them that even some of the skinniest folks are fighting the same battle. T2DM doesn't discriminate—it's an equal-opportunity nightmare. And maybe, just maybe, it's time we stopped trying to pin it all on the scale and started looking deeper.

In this book, Balanced Life, we'll delve into the often-overlooked details of body fat—both the visible fat and the fat that lurks in your blood. But that's not all. We'll explore different approaches to achieving your ideal health results based on your unique health, history, and circumstances. Whether you're underweight, healthy, overweight, or obese, there's something here for you.

The goal isn't to offer a quick fix for weight loss, but to help you understand weight management through a health-focused lens. This book is about long-term health—taking a deep dive into how you can eat and live in ways that make you feel your best.

The science may be complicated, and I get that. But don't worry— I've worked hard to break it down into digestible pieces. If you find yourself feeling overwhelmed, remember: you don't have to navigate this alone. Your doctor, the internet, and even this book are all here to help guide you to the answers you need.

This is not a handbook on how to become the next beauty queen (or king)—let's leave that to the runway models. Instead, it's about providing you with knowledge and understanding that you can apply in your own life, however you see fit.

As Mahatma Gandhi once wisely said, *"Live as if you were to die tomorrow, but learn as if you were to live forever."* Knowledge is power—but only if it's used the right way. There's no one-size-fits-all plan for maintaining a healthy weight, but with the proper education, commitment, and balance, you can achieve your health goals without sacrificing your happiness or joy along the way.

2. Benefits of a Balanced Life

2.1. Lower Your Cholesterol

LDL cholesterol, the bad boy of the cholesterol world, is always causing trouble and clogging up your arteries like a traffic jam on a Monday morning. High LDL cholesterol levels are like that friend who shows up at your party uninvited, eats all your snacks, and leaves your place in a mess. When LDL cholesterol builds up, it forms plaque, which can slowly choke off your blood vessels—a condition known as **atherosclerosis**. Congratulations, you've just earned yourself a **heart attack** if this happens in your heart. If it happens in your brain, well, enjoy the **stroke** party. It's the kind of event you really don't want to attend.

But don't worry, here comes **HDL cholesterol**, the good guy in the cholesterol world. Think of HDL as the unsung hero swooping in to remove the bad LDL cholesterol from your bloodstream and tossing it to the liver like it's a hot potato. The liver's job? Break it down and kick it out of your system.

Now, for the good news: you can give LDL cholesterol the boot by losing some weight and putting HDL cholesterol to work. A **balanced diet** is your first line of defence. If you cut down on red meat, you can lower your LDL cholesterol—because, let's face it, red meat is like the cheerleader for LDL. The more you consume, the more LDL you get. Also, ditching those fatty foods reduces the very building blocks of LDL cholesterol—kind of like cleaning out a hoarder's house.

And hey, fibre's not just for digestion—it's got a dirty little secret. Your body can't absorb it, but fibre can totally team up with cholesterol byproducts and drag them out of your system like a bouncer at the club. So, a high-fibre diet can literally help clear out the LDL party crasher.

Lastly, get off your butt and start doing some cardio. Your heart is basically a muscle that uses fat to do its job, so the harder it works, the more fat you burn. That's right, it's basically an internal fat-burning machine. Plus, cardio gets HDL into action, which then gives LDL a one-way ticket out of town. Aim for 30 minutes of cardio at least three times a week, and you'll not only lower your LDL but also keep your heart in tip-top shape, ready to handle whatever life throws at you—hopefully, not another stroke or heart attack.

2.2.   Reduce The Risk of Heart Disease

Proper weight management and regular exercise are your heart's best friends. They're like that personal trainer who helps you lose weight and keeps you out of the doctor's office. Too much weight—especially around the belly—can invite heart disease to your doorstep, and you definitely don't want that guest. On the other hand, losing weight can make your heart as happy as a cat in a sunbeam.

LDL cholesterol, the villain of the cardiovascular world, can form plaques in your arteries, clogging up the pathways that deliver blood to your heart. When your heart doesn't get enough blood, it's like trying to run a marathon on a busy sidewalk. Eventually, the heart muscle starts to wither away—slowly, but surely. It's like watching a tragic movie, but you don't want to be the one to star in it.

And speaking of slow death, bad diets can put your heart on the same track. Take **vitamin B1 (thiamine) deficiency**, for instance. It can lead to **wet beriberi**—a condition where your heart literally weakens and can fail. This is typically tied to **malnutrition** or **chronic alcoholism**, neither of which are great ways to show your heart some love.

But here's the good news: lowering LDL cholesterol and boosting HDL cholesterol can give your heart a fighting chance. By making these adjustments, you're not just extending your life—you're giving your heart a reason to keep going. So, ditch the junk, get moving, and your heart will thank you with every beat. Your heart will go from saying thumb thumb to saying thank you thank you.

2.3. Lower Blood Pressure

Elevated LDL cholesterol is like that annoying friend who takes up space and makes everything harder to deal with. First, it thickens your blood, increasing **blood viscosity**—fancy speak for making your blood feel like molasses. On top of that, LDL is busy clogging your arteries with plaque, narrowing those blood vessels, and making everything more of a struggle. The result? Strained blood vessels that can easily lead to high blood pressure. So, by lowering your LDL cholesterol, you're not just clearing out the traffic jams in your arteries but also giving your blood pressure a well-needed break.

Regular exercise and a balanced diet are like your blood's personal spa day—especially when it comes to weight management. Exercise ramps up **nitric oxide** production, which is basically a "relaxation potion" for your blood vessels. Nitric oxide helps keep those vessels nice and relaxed, allowing for smoother blood flow and, yep, lower blood pressure. It also helps your heart and lungs function better, giving you a cardiovascular upgrade that's as good as hitting the reset button. So, put down the chips, pick up the dumbbells, and let your blood pressure enjoy the peace and quiet!

2.4. Reduce The Risk of Strokes

Obesity is basically an all-access pass to a stroke waiting to happen, especially when it brings along high LDL cholesterol as its +1. When you're carrying excess weight, LDL cholesterol happily builds up in your arteries, turning them into narrow passageways. This could lead to a **serious brain malfunction**—also known as a stroke—when the blood supply to your brain is cut off. So, if you want to keep your brain functioning, losing weight is a great way to lower the odds of a stroke and boost your brain health.

But wait, there's more! If your blood pressure goes rogue and stages a coup called **malignant hypertension** (blood pressure over 180/120 mmHg), it can cause your blood to start clotting like a bad party guest who just won't leave. These clots can then hitch a ride to your brain and cause a stroke. So, besides shedding some pounds, controlling your blood pressure is key to keeping your brain and body on the up and up.

2.5. Improve Blood Flow

LDL cholesterol is like that uninvited guest who sneaks into your arteries and sets up shop, blocking blood flow to your heart and other vital organs. But don't worry—by lowering LDL cholesterol and boosting your HDL cholesterol with a balanced diet and lifestyle, you can clear out the clutter and improve blood flow, reducing the risk of heart attacks and strokes.

Exercise is your secret weapon in this battle. It strengthens your heart and helps your blood vessels work better, promoting circulation and reducing your risk of heart disease and other health issues. When your heart pumps more efficiently, it sends oxygen-rich blood to all your cells and tissues, keeping you in tip-top shape.

Exercise also works wonders for your blood vessels, **improving their elasticity and reducing inflammation**. This helps blood flow more freely and reduces your risk of circulation problems, such as **varicose veins**.

On the flip side, carrying excess weight can strain your blood vessels, causing inflammation and a condition called endothelial dysfunction that messes with blood flow. But don't panic! Losing weight and exercising regularly can help reverse this damage, improve circulation, and keep your blood vessels happy and healthy. So, lace up those sneakers and get moving—you've got this!

2.6. Reduce Inflammation

Inflammation is like that annoying, persistent problem that keeps popping up at the worst times. It's a major contributor to heart disease and many other health issues. Thankfully, HDL cholesterol is the superhero in this scenario, stepping in with its anti-inflammatory powers to fight off the bad stuff and keep you feeling better.

Obesity, unfortunately, is like inviting inflammation to the party. It raises your risk of heart disease and other complications. **Chronic inflammation**, which is your body's reaction to injury or infection, can hang around longer than you'd like and contribute to lasting problems like heart conditions. That minor heart inflammation? If left unchecked, it can sneak up on you and develop into chronic heart disease.

Chronic inflammation is even more dangerous when it brings along a dangerous guest called cancer. Inflammation can encourage cancer cells to grow and spread. But here's the good news—losing weight and exercising regularly can help turn down the volume on inflammation. Exercise doesn't just burn fat; it also boosts the production of **anti-inflammatory compounds**, giving you a full-on, holistic defence against inflammation. So, hit the gym and take control of your health—you'll look better and feel better, too.

2.7. Improve Insulin Sensitivity

Being overweight or obese messes with **insulin sensitivity**, which is your body's way of saying, *"Hey, I can't deal with all this sugar traffic—fix it!"* The solution? Ditch the extra fluff and start exercising. Turns out, burning fat and building muscle doesn't just make you look good—it makes your cells actually listen to insulin instead of ghosting it.

Insulin sensitivity is like glucose's ability to RSVP to the party in your body: the better it is, the more glucose gets invited in and stored properly. Exercise helps by producing glucose transporters, which are like the Uber drivers for sugar. They shuttle glucose straight into your cells. Without them, sugar is just awkwardly loitering in your bloodstream, wrecking the vibe.

Obesity is basically the overachiever of health risks, racking up points for Type 2 diabetes mellitus (T2DM), heart disease, and more. T2DM, for the uninitiated, is when your body either stops listening to insulin altogether (type 2) or your pancreas taps out and stops producing insulin (type 1). Losing weight and sweating it out lowers your chances of this metabolic mutiny—and makes your pancreas less likely to write its resignation letter.

Bonus points for exercise: it cranks out **glucose-transporter 4 (GT4)**, the MVP of sugar transport, and insulin-sensitive enzymes. These help keep your cells on speaking terms with insulin, reducing your risk of T2DM. So, hit the treadmill and keep your cells and sugar on good terms—because nothing screams "adulting" like managing your insulin sensitivity before it ruins the party.

2.8. Improve Mental Health

Carrying extra weight isn't just hard on your joints—it's a total buzzkill for your brain, too. Excess weight messes with your **cognitive function**, like memory and concentration, because your brain's blood vessels are busy dealing with cholesterol traffic jams instead of delivering oxygen. That's right—those LDL cholesterol plaques aren't just clogging your heart but also staging a hostile takeover in your brain's oxygen supply chain. The result? Brain fog that feels like your neurons are perpetually hungover.

But there's hope! Manage your weight, and your brain might stop acting like it's on dial-up internet. You'll boost blood flow, get more oxygen upstairs, and maybe even remember where you left your car keys.

On top of all that, obesity has a way of dragging your mental health into the gutter. **Depression** and **anxiety** love to hitch a ride on excess weight, thanks to the wrecking ball it takes to your **self-esteem** and body image. Losing weight isn't just about squeezing into your old jeans; it's about giving your mind a break from the constant soundtrack of self-criticism. Slimming down might not fix everything, but it's a solid first step toward turning your brain's pity party into something that feels a little more like a dance floor.

2.9. Improve Sexual Function and Fertility

Carrying extra weight doesn't just make your pants tight—it tightens the screws on your sex life, too. Excess pounds can tank your **libido**, turn the bedroom into a stress zone, and even mess with the plumbing downstairs. Let's break it down, shall we?

First, the mechanics: obesity causes inflammation, which chokes off blood flow like a bad traffic jam on date night. Reduced blood flow means nerves in your favourite areas might throw in the towel. Men, say hello to **erectile dysfunction**. Women, welcome to the land of desert-like conditions. Fun, right?

But wait, there's more! Those extra pounds can also trash your hormones. In women, this might mean **disrupted ovulation** and a VIP ticket to **PCOS**-ville. In men, abdominal obesity becomes the ultimate **testosterone** thief, leaving you with fewer swimmers in the fertility pool.

And the psychological sabotage? That's just the cherry on top. Low self-esteem and poor body image can leave you avoiding the mirror—and your partner. Losing weight and hitting the gym doesn't just help with stamina (yes, cardio counts as foreplay); it boosts confidence, testosterone, and your overall mojo.

As for fertility? Dropping a few pounds can get your hormones back in line, making baby-making a bit less stressful. And let's not forget the post-workout glow: **endorphins** reduce stress, anxiety, and awkwardness. So, if you've been feeling like your love life is stuck in neutral, maybe it's time to let sweat be your sexy.

2.10.   Reduce The Risk of Joint Problems

Carrying extra weight doesn't just make your knees scream for mercy; it turns your joints into a dysfunctional family reunion where nobody gets along. Here's how it plays out: the **cartilage** that's supposed to keep your bones from grinding together says, *"I quit!"* Next thing you know, it's bone-on-bone warfare, also known as **osteoarthritis**. Congrats, the family get-together of your joints just became a horror movie.

But don't despair—there's hope. Losing weight is like firing the referee back into the game. Shedding those pounds takes the pressure off your joints, and regular exercise swoops in like a superhero, strengthening muscles and bones to support the drama-riddled joints.

Mobility, too, gets a serious upgrade. Excess weight turns simple tasks—like getting out of a chair—into an Olympic event. Lose some of that extra baggage, and suddenly, you're doing cartwheels (okay, maybe just walking without flinching). Strong muscles and a lively cardiovascular system make moving around feel less like hauling a truckload of bricks.

And let's talk pain relief. Dropping the pounds isn't just good for your waistline—it's your joints' way of saying, *"Thank you for not crushing me anymore."* Plus, exercise fights inflammation like a tiny army of anti-inflammatory ninjas, reducing swelling and alleviating pain.

Flexibility also comes to the party when you start exercising. Stretching and strengthening muscles, ligaments, and joints isn't just good for your range of motion—it's the yoga equivalent of whispering sweet nothings to your body.

So, the next time your knees protest with every step, show them some love with a little weight loss and a lot of movement, which are the keys to joint happiness. It's like therapy, but cheaper—and sweatier.

2.11. Decrease Stress and Risk of Depression

Stress and obesity go together like an awkward couple at a dance—no one's having a good time, and everything feels heavier than it should. Excess weight can drag your self-esteem into the mud, leaving you staring at the mirror and wondering when your reflection became such a bully. But fear not! Exercise is here, wearing a cape made of **endorphins**.

Endorphins are like your brain's personal stash of happy juice. Hit the gym, go for a jog, or even power-walk past your problems, and these feel-good chemicals will flood your system, making stress slink away like it's just been caught stealing cookies. Add **serotonin** to the mix—your brain's mood DJ—and suddenly, life's playlist has a lot more bangers.

Self-esteem and body image also get a major glow-up when you shed those extra pounds. Losing weight isn't just about looking good in selfies (though that helps); it's about walking into a room like you own it. Confidence skyrockets when your body feels stronger, fitter, and less like it's conspiring against you.

As for depression, it's no match for endorphins and **brain-derived neurotrophic factor** (BDNF)—the unsung hero of your neural network. BDNF is like Miracle-Gro for your brain, keeping your neurons bubbly and your mood sunny.

And let's not forget about relaxation. Stress hormones take a nosedive when you embrace exercise or deep-breathing techniques. Suddenly, you're the chilliest person in the room, radiating calm vibes while everyone else is losing their minds over deadlines and existential crises.

So, if you're tired of stress sitting on your calorie-gifted behind like a particularly grumpy cat, grab your sneakers and get moving. Your brain, body, and sanity will thank you—preferably with a round of applause and a well-earned slice of serotonin pie.

2.12. Improve Sleep Quality

Carrying extra weight can turn your nights into a game of "How Many Sheep Can I Count Before I Lose It?" Excess weight often invites **snoring**, **restless leg syndrome**, and **insomnia** to crash your nightly slumber party, leaving you groggy and ready to fight your alarm clock come morning. But don't despair—weight loss and exercise can rescue your sleep like the hero it's meant to be.

First up, inflammation. Excess weight stirs up inflammation like a bad soap opera villain, but shedding pounds helps cool that drama, letting your body (and brain) finally get some peace and quiet. Plus, exercise boosts endorphins, which are like nature's bedtime lullaby—relaxing you enough to stop doom-scrolling and actually close your eyes.

Then there's **melatonin**, your sleep hormone BFF. Regular exercise gently nudges melatonin into production, helping regulate your sleep cycle like a finely tuned Swiss watch. Just don't overdo the late-night workouts—spiking cortisol levels too close to bedtime might leave you lying awake, thinking about everything you ever said in middle school.

Let's not ignore sleep saboteurs like snoring or restless leg syndrome. Losing weight can quiet that midnight chainsaw impersonation (your partner will thank you) and calm those jittery legs, making your bed a sanctuary rather than a battleground.

Finally, remember that good sleep isn't just about avoiding morning grumpiness—it's essential for overall health and sanity. So, trade the late-night snacks for some light stretching, lace up those running shoes, and tell sleepless nights to take a hike.

2.13.   Regulate Hormone Levels

Obesity's connection to cancer is like that one messy friend who always stirs up trouble at the party—it's uninvited, unwanted, and hard to ignore. Extra weight throws your hormones into chaos, creating a playground for certain cancers to thrive. But there's good news: ditching the excess baggage and embracing exercise can help kick that freeloading douchebag to the curb.

For starters, exercise acts like your body's hormone whisperer. By promoting the production of **estrogen-metabolizing enzymes**, it helps keep **hormone-sensitive cancers**, like breast cancer, from setting up shop. Think of it as Marie Kondo-ing your internal system—if the hormone isn't sparking joy, it gets shown the door.

Then there's **insulin and IGF-1**, the cancer-enabling duo. These two troublemakers are linked to an increased risk of breast cancer. Regular workouts reduce their levels, essentially cutting off cancer's power supply. It's like turning off the Wi-Fi on that one freeloading neighbour who keeps stealing your signal.

And don't forget inflammation. Excess weight stirs it up like a bad reality show, but weight loss and exercise can calm things down, giving your body the fighting chance it deserves.

So, if your hormones are acting like hormonal teenagers, crank up the cardio and let exercise restore some balance. Not only will it help reduce cancer risks, but it also gives you a great excuse to buy more athleisure wear—because nothing says *"I'm fighting cancer risk"* like a new pair of leggings.

2.14. Improve Immune Function

Exercise is like your immune system's personal trainer, whipping it into shape and keeping it ready to fight off life's heavyweights— like infections, diseases, and even cancer. Picture your immune cells in tiny sweatbands, doing push-ups every time you hit the gym.

For starters, working out boosts the production of antibodies and immune cells like **T cells and natural killer cells**. These are your body's bouncers, kicking out intruders and troublemakers before they cause chaos. Think of them as the nightclub security guards, but for your bloodstream.

And let's talk about inflammation—because nothing ruins a good immune system party like a bunch of inflamed tissues showing up uninvited. Regular exercise acts as the anti-inflammatory bouncer, calming the chaos and keeping things under control so your immune system can focus on its main gig: protecting you.

So, the next time you're dragging yourself to a workout, remember: you're not just sweating for better abs or a smaller waistline—you're giving your immune system the Rocky Balboa training montage it deserves. And who doesn't want an immune system that's ready to yell, *"Yo, infection, you're going down!"?*

2.15. Improve Your Energy Levels

Carrying extra weight is like wearing a heavy backpack you never asked for—every activity feels like a hike up Mount Everest. This constant strain drains your energy faster than an old smartphone battery with a dozen apps running in the background.

Dropping those extra pounds can help you shed more than just weight—it's like ditching the unnecessary luggage. Suddenly, climbing stairs doesn't feel like scaling Mount Kilimanjaro, and bending down to tie your shoes doesn't require a recovery period.

Pair that with exercise, and you've got a double whammy of awesomeness. Your body gets better at burning calories and managing energy, like upgrading from a rusty old pinto to a fuel-efficient modern hybrid. Plus, exercise gives you a hit of endorphins—the feel-good chemicals that boost your mood and slap fatigue in the face.

So, lose weight, gain energy, and start living like someone who finally ditched the backpack for a jetpack.

Remember that no magic pill or miracle diet exists for weight management and exercise. If there were, we'd all be living on pizza and still somehow rocking six-packs. The key is a healthy, sustainable approach that doesn't involve drastic measures or extreme fads.

Team up with a healthcare professional to map out a plan that suits you. This isn't about turning your life into a boot camp—it's about setting reasonable goals, tracking your progress, and making changes that you can maintain without crying into a kale salad every night.

Start small with a healthy diet and sprinkle in some exercise, but don't expect overnight results. This is a long-term relationship you're building with your body, not a one-night stand. Stick with it, and you'll reap the rewards of better energy levels and a sustainable weight that doesn't require you to starve yourself or live in the gym.

3.   Getting Started

3.1.   Nature Vs Nurture

Scientists, statisticians, and even the occasional economist agree that life tends to follow a bell curve—because, of course, the universe just had to organize itself like a high school math lesson. This Gaussian distribution means most of us get crammed into the "meh, average" category, while a lucky few get to be outliers, living it up at the extremes (or, you know, just living in their weird little corners of reality).

Take height, for example. About 80% of North American men over 18 are between 5'5" and 6'. They're the middle ground—the human equivalent of vanilla ice cream. The remaining 20%? They're the real winners of the genetic lottery... or losers, depending on whether they're ducking through doorframes or shopping in the kids' section. Life's bell curve: the universe's way of saying, *"You'll probably be fine, but don't get your hopes up."*

Another classic example of the bell curve is the IQ distribution. Around 95% of people score between 70 and 130, comfortably in the middle of "functional human" territory. The top 2.5% above 130 are solving quantum physics equations for fun, while the bottom 2.5% below 70 are probably still trying to figure out how the toaster works. Honestly, who's living the better life there is up for debate.

Then there's birth weight. Most babies are born at a healthy average weight, neatly conforming to the bell curve. But fast forward a few decades, and suddenly, half of those adorable, chubby-cheeked newborns have become adult versions of walking potatoes. If birth weight stats carried through to adulthood, we'd have just as many heavy babies as obese adults. But no, life said, *"Let's shake things up and throw in fast food, stress, and Netflix binges."* The bell curve didn't stand a chance.

Over the years, there's been a lot of chatter about a "genetic predisposition" to obesity. Sounds fancy, right? It's like your DNA is secretly conspiring to make you fail at buttoning your jeans. But here's the twist: it's never actually been proven scientifically. Sure, genetics might load the gun, but diet, lifestyle, and binge-watching every season of Friends and Everybody Loves Raymond pull the trigger.

Let's play a little game of cat comparison. Wild cats in developing and developed countries weigh roughly the same, living their lives hunting, climbing trees, and judging humans from afar. But house cats? Oh boy. In developed countries, they're living the dream: endless kibble, no predators, and the occasional stolen slice of pizza. Boom—sometimes twice the weight of their counterparts in less cushy environments. It's not genetics; it's nurture—or, in this case, over-nurture.

Genetics isn't a life sentence—it's more like a memo. If your parents had the "big-boned" DNA instructions, they might pass those along. But that doesn't mean you're destined to star in The Biggest Loser. It's just a probability, not a prophecy. Think of your DNA as a recipe—you can tweak it with your own ingredients, like kale, a treadmill, and the willpower to ignore that 2 a.m. pizza craving.

So, are you doomed to carry your parents' extra baggage if they were/are overweight? Nope. Even if they hand you the genetic manual for "Chunky 101," it's up to you whether you follow it or write a new chapter titled "Skinny Genes and Salad Dreams."

Mutations sound like something straight out of a superhero origin story, but in real life? They're more like the plot twist no one asked for. The good news? Most dangerous mutations don't make it past the reproductive finish line. If they do, the resulting offspring typically won't stick around long enough to find out the meaning of a credit score. Faulty DNA may exist, but it's rarely the direct cause of your body's structure looking like a Picasso painting.

That said, faulty genes can make you more vulnerable to environmental factors—like bad air, bad habits, or bad decisions (looking at you, triple bacon cheeseburger with extra fries and a milkshake). **Genetic diseases**? They're often the messy offspring of vulnerable DNA meeting a toxic environment. Think of it as a bad Tinder match, but for your health.

Now, if someone tries to argue that your ever-expanding waistline is thanks to mom and dad's faulty genes, here's the kicker: it's almost impossible to prove scientifically. DNA might play a role, but so does your unrelenting love affair with fast food. Ultimately, whether your genes or triple cheeseburgers got you here, the real issue is that you're carrying extra weight—and not the philosophical kind.

When the words "live healthier" come up, some people immediately hear, *"Lose weight or die trying."* Cue the internal meltdown. That overwhelming thought alone is enough to drive them straight back to the cookie jar. The truth is, focusing on the endgame—shedding X pounds—is about as helpful as telling someone to "just be rich." Spoiler alert: it's not.

Instead, baby steps are your best friend. Please don't make it about the number on the scale; make it about the wins you can actually see. Lowering cholesterol? Check. Blood sugar that won't have your pancreas dialling 911? Double check. Blood pressure not mimicking a volcano about to erupt? Gold star. Or even simpler— try eating fewer processed atrocities masquerading as food or finding time to move more than just your thumbs.

This approach isn't just common sense; psychologists back it up. Scaring smokers with lung cancer stats rarely works. But tell them their habit gives them dragon breath, teeth straight out of a horror flick, and skin that could double as parchment? Suddenly, they're all ears. The same principle applies to weight loss. Forget about dropping a hundred pounds—how about just building the stamina to vacuum your bedroom without sounding like a dying walrus or maintaining the flexibility to tie your shoes without turning it into an Olympic event?

And for the love of stretch pants, don't aim for rapid weight loss. If you're shedding more than 1% of your body weight a week, you're either a contestant on a reality show or ignoring all reasonable advice. Weight management isn't a sprint; it's a slow, often sweaty, sometimes snack-filled marathon. So, lace up, pace yourself, and maybe leave the scale alone for a while.

3.2. Hard vs Impossible

Someone once said, "No one trips over mountains; it's the tiny pebbles that send you face-planting." And honestly, isn't that the truth? The trick is to tackle those pesky pebbles one at a time. Before you know it, you'll look back and realize you've conquered the whole mountain—without a single dramatic tumble. Well, maybe just a few.

It's the same idea behind the old saying, "A journey of a thousand miles begins with one step." Sure, it's a cliché, but clichés stick around for a reason—they work. Breaking that thousand-mile trek into bite-sized pieces makes it less daunting. Take one step, then another, and suddenly, you're a mile in. Celebrate that mile! Then rinse, repeat, and before long, you'll be at mile 1,000, wondering why you ever stressed about it in the first place.

The secret isn't obsessing over the entire journey—it's focusing on what's right in front of you. Because, let's be honest, the thought of a thousand miles is enough to make anyone lie down and nap. But a single step? That's doable. One pebble at a time, one mile at a time—that's how you cross mountains, finish marathons, or even clean out your junk drawer.

At least 30% of people in the Western world are obese or morbidly obese, with some experts predicting that figure could balloon to over 50% in the coming decades. That means half of us might be rolling down the street like human bowling balls—and hey, maybe someone out there is hoping to turn it into a world record. Dream big, right?

But let's face it: life isn't simple. Sure, there are those infuriating people who make everything look easy. Whether they're dropping 50 pounds, running a marathon, or assembling IKEA furniture without swearing, they make the rest of us feel like uncoordinated toddlers trying to use chopsticks.

What we don't see is the sheer blood, sweat, and probably a few tears they poured into their success. Behind every seemingly effortless achievement lies a mountain of preparation, training, and trial and error. Athletes? They didn't just roll out of bed with six-packs. Machines? Someone stayed up all night perfecting those gears. Furniture? Okay, let's not give IKEA too much credit, but you get the idea.

The point is that most of us only see the final, polished result—not the chaos, missteps, and caffeine-fuelled breakdowns that came before it. So, if you're struggling to start your own journey—weight loss or otherwise—remember this: even the masters had their messy beginnings.

Even though Olympic sprinters are on the track for about 10 glorious seconds, the real show happens in the months and years of training—hours upon hours of sweat, blisters, and regrettable protein shakes. That's the price they pay for a moment of glory, and honestly, it's the same deal with getting the body you want. Think of your dream physique as your personal Olympic event, minus the cheering crowd (or maybe with a few, if you've got supportive pets).

When it comes to weight management or healthier living, don't get caught up fantasizing about your future as a human mannequin or a blood pressure reading that doesn't scare your doctor. Instead, start by getting to know yourself. What are your strengths? Weaknesses? Why do you want to do this? Is it for better health, to make your ex jealous, or just to stop wheezing while walking upstairs? Whatever it is, own it.

Once you've figured that out, it's time to set goals. And not just any goals—S.M.A.R.T. ones: Specific, Measurable, Achievable,

Realistic, and Time-sensitive. In other words, no *"I want to look like a Marvel superhero by next Tuesday."* Start small, like *"I will walk 20 minutes a day,"* and build from there. Rome wasn't built in a day, nor is your dream body. But hey, at least Rome didn't have to deal with kale smoothies.

Saying you want to drop 100 pounds in six months is like saying you want to become a brain surgeon by binge-watching medical dramas—it's technically a plan, but it's got disaster written all over it. Sure, the goal is specific and measurable, but let's be honest— it's about as achievable and realistic as Yokozuna running a marathon without training. Even if you could pull it off, it wouldn't be healthy. Losing that much weight that fast is practically a health crisis in itself, paving the way to **gallstones**, **pancreatitis**, and, ironically, gaining back every pound (plus a few extras) when you inevitably crash.

Here's the hard truth: slow and steady wins the race, especially when it comes to weight loss. The sweet spot is no more than 1% of your body weight per week—enough to make progress without turning your body into a walking science experiment. People who pace themselves keep the weight off and build habits that stick around longer than a New Year's resolution.

So, ditch the quick-fix mindset. This is a marathon, not a sprint— and unlike a marathon, you don't need special shoes or a medal at the end. Just healthier habits, one week at a time.

When the goal is to walk 10 kilometres a day, you don't start by strapping on a Fitbit and declaring yourself the next Forrest Gump. No, you begin humbly—perhaps by strolling to the fridge and back (but please don't open the fridge!). If that's your comfortable distance, own it. Maybe it's 400 metres instead. Walk it. Jot it down. Then rinse and repeat until you're crushing those 400 metres like it's nothing. Next week? Go for 600 metres. The week after? A kilometre. Before you know it, you'll be the 10-kilometre champ of your neighbourhood mall walkers.

The same logic applies to pushups. If doing one pushup feels like trying to bench-press a car, don't worry. Start on your knees—embrace the "half-pushup." Can't manage that either? Lean on a wall and push back like you're politely rejecting an awkward hug. Find your starting point, no matter how basic, and work from there.

Once you can do one pushup, resist the temptation to crank out 20 immediately. You're not auditioning for an action movie montage. Do one, then rest. Do another. Rest again. Build up gradually, like stacking Lego bricks—one piece at a time, but without the foot-stabbing hazard.

The secret sauce here? Patience. Rome wasn't built in a day, and neither is a fitness routine. Be kind to your body. Small wins add up over time; before you know it, you'll hit that big achievement you set out for. Bonus: you'll get there without pulling a muscle or needing an embarrassing trip to the ER.

4. The Normal

4.1. The Fat Cell

Fat cells are the tiny energy hoarders squatting rent-free in your body, waiting for their chance to shine. These little suckers, also known as **adipocytes**, have been humanity's ride-or-die survival mechanism for millions of years. Back in the hunter-gatherer days, when food was like a seasonal lottery, fat cells were the ultimate life hack. Feast hard, store the energy, and ride out the famine like a biological prepper with a well-stocked bunker.

Fast forward to today, where the closest thing to a famine is running out of snacks during a Netflix binge. Fat cells, bless their loyal little nuclei, haven't caught on that times have changed. They're still stockpiling calories like there's a breadline around the corner, but instead of saving us from starvation, they're making sure we can't squeeze into our favourite jeans.

Modern feasting is less about surviving and more about seeing how much cheese you can legally put on a pizza. But instead of using that stored energy to outrun predators or survive winter, most of us just sit there, conserving so much energy we can barely stand up without needing a snack.

The environmental impact? Oh, it's a buffet of consequences. Food production, water, and energy usage skyrocket to sustain our energy-hoarding habits. Basically, the planet's doing burpees to support our endless calorie collection, and it's starting to look pretty winded. So, the next time you reach for that second dessert, remember that your fat cells are already busy preparing for an apocalypse that's never coming.

These overachievers of the cellular world are like that friend who insists on hoarding toilet paper during a sale, except he lives alone but is shopping for a family of ten with perpetual diarrhea. Sure, they've got all the usual cell parts like a nucleus and cytoplasm, but their pièce de résistance is a whopping 90% fat reservoir. Talk about committing to the role.

Medically speaking, fat cells are the celebrities of obesity studies, and not the glamorous kind. When these little energy hoarders get too ambitious, they tip the scales—literally—into obesity territory. That's when things start to go sideways, with an increased risk of heart disease, T2DM, and cancers. It's like your fat cells threw a house party and forgot to clean up, leaving you with long-term consequences. Thanks, guys.

Socially, fat cells have also stirred up drama. Obesity is often treated like a scarlet letter, with society pinning everything from laziness to poor life choices on anyone carrying extra weight. This stigma isn't just mean-spirited—it's damaging, leading to isolation, discrimination, and a steady stream of sad violin music in the lives of those affected.

The solution? Balance. A healthy diet, some movement (no, not just to the fridge), and a bit of self-love. While fat cells are unique, they're not your enemy—they are just misunderstood overachievers who need a bit of management. Let's keep them busy without letting them take over the show, shall we?

By the tender age of seven, your body has already decided how many of these little calorie hoarders you'll be stuck with. After that, they only expand, like party balloons with a bottomless helium tank. Occasionally, when they outgrow their accommodations, they start inviting friends over. That's right— new fat cells show up, ready to turn your calorie surplus into a long-term commitment.

Preschool and puberty are the golden years for fat cell recruitment. Preschool is particularly risky because your body's still assembling its lifelong fat cell squad. It's like handing a toddler the keys to a candy store and saying, *"Go nuts."* At least during puberty, hormones give teenagers enough energy to burn off some of those extra calories—assuming they're not glued to a screen, developing thumbs of steel.

Parents, here's the catch: Kids are on a "see-food" diet during these critical growth spurts. If they see it, they'll eat it. It's your mission to make sure the menu skews more toward salad and less toward triple cheeseburgers. Because those extra nuggets aren't just temporary—they're invitations for new fat cells to crash the party, and trust me, they're not leaving anytime soon.

Next time your kid reaches for a snack, make sure it's something green and less likely to start a lifelong battle of expansion. After all, preventing a fat cell uprising is easier than staging a revolution later.

Fat cells, nature's rubber-band hoarders, are indeed the gift that keeps on giving—especially if you keep feeding them. Let's break it down using everyone's favourite colourful analogy: Skittles. Imagine your fat cell membrane as a perfect circle made of Skittles, each piece representing a part of that fat-storing barrier. Add one Skittle to the radius of the membrane, and not only does the perimeter grow, but the area—where the fat reserves live—expands exponentially.

For the naturally skinny folks (the ones who complain about needing extra snacks and blankets, bless their oblivious hearts), assuming a perfect circle, a radius of 5 Skittles gives us a perimeter of 31 Skittles and an area of 79 $Skittles^2$. Adding one Skittle to the radius gives a perimeter of 38 Skittles and an area of 113 $Skittles^2$, which is like upgrading from a kiddie pool to a slightly larger kiddie pool. That's a 20% increase in perimeter (membrane size) and 44% in area (fat reservoirs). This demonstrates the power of increased membrane size in determining how many more excess calories your fat cells can store. However, the body works hard to make that one extra Skittle, so it's no walk in the park for them to gain weight.

Now, for our friends who've already amassed a fat cell empire, adding a single Skittle to their already colossal circle is like expanding an Olympic-sized pool. Assuming a radius of 20 Skittles gives us a perimeter of 126 Skittles and an area of 1,257 $Skittles^2$. Adding one Skittle to the radius gives a perimeter of 132

Skittles and an area of 1,385 Skittles^2.

While that's only an increase of 5% in perimeter (membrane size) and 10% in the area (fat reservoirs), that one annoying Skittle radius increased the fat reservoirs by 128 skittles^2 in Ms. Big and Fabulous. The same lone Skittle in Skinny Joe only increased the fat reservoir by 35 skittles^2. That's nearly 3 times the weight gain in the Fluffy Folks compared to Ultra Featherweight Champs with the same increase in the size of the fat cell membrane. The fat cells of Fluffy Folks are like seasoned hoarders finding new closets to stuff.

But here's the kicker: losing weight flips the script. Fat cells don't want to shed their precious membrane easily. First, they'll dump the reserves before reluctantly shrinking the membrane. This means that obese individuals have to work nearly three times harder to burn off that one Skittle's worth of fat compared to their underweight counterparts.

Fat cells are both overachievers and stubborn jerks. They make gaining weight absurdly efficient when you're bigger but demand Herculean effort to downsize. So, the next time someone tells you, *"It's just one cookie,"* remember: that's one Skittle closer to your fat cells planning an expansion.

Fat cells are like overzealous landlords: even when the tenants (fat reserves) leave, they refuse to downsize their mansions (cell membranes). Rapidly losing weight drains the reserves, but those oversized membranes stick around, ready to welcome back the calorie tenants at the first glimpse of a cheesecake. This explains why people who shed pounds too quickly often gain it all back just as fast—**yo-yo dieting** at its finest.

Here's another kicker: when the reserves are gone, but the mansion still stands, it's way easier to refill those rooms with more fat. If, however, you manage to shrink the mansion itself (the cell membrane) along with the reserves, your body faces a major renovation bill just to start hoarding again. Making new membranes is a time-consuming, energy-sucking process—

basically the biological equivalent of building a skyscraper from scratch.

For those taking the slow and steady route, congrats! You're effectively bulldozing the fat mansions down to studio apartments. This makes it much harder for your body to pack on the pounds again, which is why gradual weight loss is far more sustainable.

Now, let's talk pregnancy—because fat cells, like in-laws, never miss a chance to overstay their welcome. Overweight women often find their fat cells gleefully hoarding reserves during pregnancy, using the "eating for two" excuse to expand their membranes even further. Post-baby, these fat cells don't just wave goodbye. Instead, they're practically begging for dessert to refill their reserves. This makes losing baby weight an uphill battle, especially when those oversized membranes are still lingering like the world's most persistent houseguest. More about this in Chapter 6.

Fat cells are clingy, dramatic, and bad at letting go. Please treat them with caution and maybe hide the snacks.

4.2.   Calories and Energy Storage

Calories are the tiny units of energy that simultaneously fuel your life and ruin your pants. One calorie is equal to 4.182 joules, which means even your snack regrets are rooted in science. For context, it takes 4.182 joules to raise the temperature of 1 gram of water by 1°C—ironically, the same energy required to make your guilt burn hotter when you eat that extra slice of cake.

Your body puts these calories to work, powering activities like walking, talking, and scrolling endlessly on your phone. Together, all these functions form your Daily Energy Expenditure (D.E.E.). But when you don't burn all the energy you consume, your body says, *"No problem, we'll save it for later!"* and stashes it away— mostly in fat cells and a little bit in glycogen stores, like a biological rainy-day fund.

Let's talk adipose tissue, the body's favourite fat-stashing expert. Made up of adipocytes, this tissue doubles as both your emergency energy bank and a built-in bubble wrap for your organs. It's distributed all over—under your skin, around your organs, and in those delightful "specialized fat depot areas" like your hips, thighs, and abdomen. These areas are where weight gain first makes its unwelcome debut, turning your jeans into body armour.

But adipose tissue isn't all bad. Beyond making your winter coat optional, it provides cushioning and insulation, protecting your organs from physical and environmental damage. So, the next time you catch sight of your "specialized fat depot areas" in the mirror, just remember—they're really your body's way of saying, *"You're welcome for the protection."*

Food is energy—or, as your body sees it, a currency that gets hoarded like it's prepping for an apocalyptic famine. First, it stores energy as **liver glycogen** (think of this as your body's wallet), then as **muscle glycogen** (your personal savings), and finally as fat in your adipose tissue (the under-mattress stash of shame). When your body needs energy, it raids your bloodstream for glucose first—like checking the couch cushions for spare change. Once that runs out, it taps into the liver's reserves.

If you've really overdone it on the treadmill or the apocalypse actually arrives, your body reluctantly heads for the fat stores. Each molecule of body fat is a **triglyceride**—three **fatty acids** and one **glycerol** combo. Break one down, and the glycerol goes to work, fuelling essential biochemical processes. The fatty acids, however, get sent to your heart, which, by the way, only accepts fatty acids as payment. Your heart is like the hipster coffee shop of organs— *"Sorry, we don't take cash, just artisanal fats."*

But there's a catch: break down too many triglycerides too fast that your heart can't keep up, and your bloodstream becomes a clogged highway of fatty acids, your body's version of a five-alarm fire. Prolonged starvation adds a dark twist—your liver starts converting those fatty acids into ketones, the brain's version of survival rations. It's like forcing your brain to survive on ramen noodles: effective, but let's not make it a habit. This is where the keto diet comes from, but don't be fooled because it is catfishing you.

Meanwhile, muscle glycogen smugly keeps itself off-limits to the rest of your body, a selfish trust fund of energy for your muscles only.

In the grand scheme of things, your body is an obsessive accountant. Overeat, and it pads your fat reserves like a paranoid hoarder. Eat too little, and it downsizes everything except your existential dread. Moderation is key unless you enjoy the thrill of extreme budgeting with your calories—and the inevitable consequence of your pants becoming either parachutes or tourniquets.

Exercise is the great equalizer—it's how you convince your body to part with its cherished stash of excess calories. Physical activity burns through those reserves, helping you stay lean and mean. Meanwhile, a sedentary lifestyle does the opposite, turning you into a calorie-storage facility with a Hulu subscription.

The dangers of overeating are common knowledge: extra calories lead to weight gain, health problems, and the existential crisis of outgrowing your favourite jeans. But eating too few calories? That's like trying to run a marathon on fumes—it leads to malnutrition, fatigue, and your body giving you the middle finger in the form of health problems.

Social and cultural factors also love to meddle in how we see calories. Some folks treat them like a bank account—saving them up for cheat days—while others behave like every meal is a jackpot waiting to be cashed in. Taken to extremes, you get the dark comedy of life: **crash dieting** or compulsive overexercising on one side, and all-you-can-eat buffet loyalty cards on the other. Both are recipes for disaster—just ask your metabolism, which hates extremes more than it hates fad diets.

Moderation is the unsung hero, but let's be honest, it's about as exciting as lukewarm tea. Still, it's the key to avoiding a lifetime of yo-yo dieting, energy crashes, and judgmental scales.

4.3. Hormones and Normal Physiology

Weight gain and weight loss? It's like a high-stakes game of hormones and physiology, where everything's trying to work against you. It's like a twisted reality show, but you're just trying to fit into your jeans instead of winning a million bucks. Let's dive into the behind-the-scenes drama that these hormones create.

4.3.1. Hormones

Insulin: Insulin is like that overzealous bouncer at the club, making sure all the glucose in your bloodstream gets into the cells where it can either get to work or party as fat. If your insulin's working overtime, you're likely looking at a fat storage binge. Too much glucose? Too much insulin. That means your fat cells are opening their doors to every glucose molecule seeking a place to party. If insulin's low, however, fat cells are less interested in hosting a party and more about turning down the music—aka releasing stored energy for weight loss.

Eating carbs? Oh, get ready for an insulin spike like your grandma's blood pressure after she finds out her retirement funds are going to a "daughter-in-law she always despised." That carb-heavy meal hits your bloodstream like a sugar bomb, spiking insulin and locking away calories like they're going out of style. Frequent carb binges? You're keeping insulin levels at VIP status—hello, weight gain.

Leptin: Leptin, produced by your fat cells, is like the body's personal trainer. It says, *"Hey, you've got enough fat stored. Maybe ease up on the snacks."* When you're lean, leptin's all chill, reducing your appetite and revving up your metabolism. But, if you're carrying extra weight, leptin starts throwing temper tantrums—aka, resistance. It's like the body's way of saying, *"Oh, you're not listening to me? Fine, I'll make you eat more and burn less!"* Result? Weight gain. Thanks, leptin, you had one job.

Cortisol: Cortisol is your stress hormone, like that cranky boss who's always yelling, *"DO MORE!"* But when cortisol's constantly elevated because you're stressed (hello, life), your body goes into hoarding mode. Suddenly, you're craving comfort food and not doing yourself any favours. High cortisol can make you feel like a hamster on a wheel, gaining weight, especially around your face and belly. If the cortisol party lasts too long, you might even get **Cushing's syndrome**, which brings the fun of weight gain, mood swings, and high blood pressure. Cool, right?

Ghrelin: Ghrelin is your stomach's way of saying, *"Hey, remember me? I'm hungry!"* When you're hungry, ghrelin throws a tantrum, spiking your appetite and pushing you to eat everything in sight. It's also the little hormone that likes to hang out with **growth hormone**, which can get involved in fat metabolism. If only ghrelin could stay quiet when you're trying to ignore that extra slice of cake. But no, it's like the voice of your stomach saying, *"Eat it, you know you want to."*

Thyroid hormone: The thyroid is like the quiet, nerdy student in class who keeps the whole metabolism party going. If it's slacking off (**hypothyroidism**), you'll struggle to burn calories, making it harder to lose weight. Too hyperactive (**hyperthyroidism**), and you're burning calories like a furnace—and good luck keeping that weight on. Either way, you've got a hormonal rollercoaster, with your metabolism as the amusement park.

Your body is a complex web of hormonal influencers, each playing a role in the epic saga of weight regulation. It's a mix of the good, the bad, and the downright frustrating. Eat too much, and your insulin is the villain; eat too little, and your metabolism is on strike. You can't win either way, can you?

4.3.2.   Normal Physiology

Metabolism is the silent force working behind the scenes, either sabotaging your attempts to fit into those jeans or playing along like a well-behaved puppy. Let's talk about how it all works, and trust me, it's not as simple as just eating a salad and calling it a day.

4.3.2.1.   Basal Metabolic Rate (BMR)

Your BMR is the energy your body burns just to keep you alive while you're doing absolutely nothing—because, apparently, your body doesn't take days off. This includes keeping your heart beating, your lungs breathing, and your liver doing its best impression of a 24/7 detox centre. The trouble is, the older you get, the less your body wants to cooperate. BMR peaks in your 20s (yes, that was the time when you could eat pizza like it was a sport), and then it slowly starts taking a nap. As you age, your muscles start packing up and moving out, leaving behind more fat, and making your metabolism sloooow to a crawl. Congratulations, you've hit your 30s!

4.3.2.2.   Hormones

Hormones—let's be honest, they're basically the drama queens of your body. One minute, they're telling you to eat an entire cake, and the next, they're slowing your metabolism down just because you've hit 35. As testosterone and growth hormone levels start to drop with age, goodbye muscle mass, hello sluggish metabolism. Men, those lucky devils, tend to have more muscle mass, which helps keep their metabolism humming along. Meanwhile, women—well, they've got the short end of the stick with more body fat, which is basically just a lazy tissue that doesn't burn many calories. So, good luck with that.

4.3.2.3.   Height

Apparently, being tall is more than just a reason to reach the top shelf; it's also an energy burn bonus. Taller folks have a higher

BMR because their bodies have more organs, tissues, and bones to keep alive. It's like their bodies are running a marathon just by existing. Meanwhile, shorter people are like, *"Hey, I don't need to burn as many calories because I've got fewer things to keep alive,"* and just chill out. In the grand scheme of things, height really is more than just a way to look over everyone at concerts.

4.3.2.4.   Daily Energy Expenditure (DEE)

Now, BMR is great and all, but let's talk about how much energy you burn when you actually do something besides doomscrolling on your phone. That's where DEE comes in. This is the grand total of your calorie-burning activities, including physical exercise and even just existing (BMR is the base rate, after all). If you're an athlete, lucky you! You get a higher energy requirement (we'll all pretend not to be jealous). But if you're just rolling through life on a sedentary lifestyle, well, your DEE is going to be a little on the sad side.

DEE = 24 * weight (kg) * PAR (Physical Activity Ratio)

PAR = 1.3 for sedentary; 1.5 for active living; 1.7 for pro or semi-pro athletes

For example:

- A 220-pound (100kg) man who never gets off the couch (PAR = 1.3) will need 3,120 calories to maintain his weight. His metabolism is like that of a lazy teenager.
- A 110-pound (50kg) female sprinter (PAR = 1.7)? She only needs 2,040 calories to stay at her current weight because her metabolism is doing full-on Olympic-level work 24/7.

Want to calculate your own DEE? Go ahead, use the formula like a math whiz.

And let's face it: the more sedentary you are, the less you'll burn, and the more you eat, the more likely you'll pack on those extra pounds—like your metabolism is playing the world's slowest game of catch-up. Enjoy.

4.4. Balanced Diet

A balanced diet isn't just some lofty goal or a Pinterest recipe—it's your body's survival kit. The trick is getting the right mix of foods so your body doesn't go into crisis mode. You know, those days when you're eating pizza at 2 a.m. because you couldn't bother to get a real meal. But don't worry, let's break it down and make sure you understand what each nutrient does without giving you a panic attack about how you ate three donuts today.

4.4.1. Carbohydrates: The Sweet and Starchy Energy Boost

Carbs are basically your body's fuel. Think of them like the gas in your car—without them, you're just sitting in traffic, stalled. You get carbs from grains, fruits, veggies, and legumes. But not all carbs are created equal.

- **Simple Carbs**: These are the fast food of the carb world. We're talking candy, sweet drinks, and fruit juice. They give you an energy spike, but let's be honest, they're like that one friend who leaves a mess and doesn't stick around for cleanup.
- **Complex Carbs**: These are the reliable, hardworking types—grains, legumes, potatoes. They provide you with sustained energy so you don't crash after a sugar high and end up wondering where your day went. Aim for a good mix of both so you can live your best life without being in a constant battle between *"I want cake"* and *"I need to be functional."*

4.4.2. Proteins: The Body's Bricklayers

Proteins are the builders of your body. Without them, your body would be a pile of mush. You get proteins from meat, fish, poultry, eggs, legumes, nuts, and seeds. They break down into **amino acids**, which are like the bricks in a house. There are **essential** amino acids (which your body can't make, so you need to eat them) and non-essential ones (your body can whip these up like it's making a smoothie).

It's like assembling a team of construction workers. Make sure you get a variety of protein sources so your body doesn't look like it was built by a cheap contractor.

4.4.3. Fats: The Unsung Heroes (or Villains?)

Fats are like that friend you're unsure whether you love or hate. They're great at absorbing vitamins and giving you energy, but too much of them, and you'll find yourself needing a nap just after walking to the fridge. Fats come in different varieties:

- Saturated Fats: Found in animal products and tropical oils. They're like that guy who drinks all your beer at a party, and if you let him stick around too long, he might also punch you.
- Monounsaturated and Polyunsaturated Fats: These are the heart-healthy fats from plants. They help keep your cholesterol in check, making them the responsible, calm friends at the party.

So, be wise—invite the good fats over, but don't let them overstay their welcome.

4.4.4. Vitamins: Tiny But Mighty Superheroes

Vitamins are like the sidekicks of your health, and they come in two types:

- Fat-Soluble Vitamins (A, D, E, K): These are your backup crew. They're stored in your liver and fatty tissues and don't need to be taken daily. They're like the vitamins that keep things running smoothly behind the scenes.
- Water-Soluble Vitamins (B's and C): These must be replen-

ished daily because your body doesn't have the luxury of hoarding them. It's like the vitamins are on a daily schedule, showing up to work whether you're ready or not.

If you're looking for them, you can find them in fruits, vegetables, and whole grains—because what else are they going to do with their powers but make you feel fabulous?

4.4.5. Minerals: The Body's Secret Weapon

Minerals are like the quiet, reliable people who do all the heavy lifting without asking for credit. These little guys help with everything from bone health to immune function. They come in two categories:

- Major Minerals: These are the big hitters—sodium, calcium, phosphorus, and magnesium. They're the ones that keep your bones strong and your heart beating. Get them from nuts, seeds, and leafy greens.
- Trace Minerals: These might not be as famous, but they're still important—iron, zinc, copper, iodine. They help with things like metabolism and immune function.

Without them, your body would fall apart faster than a cheap chair from a discount store.

Sure, it'd be great if you could just have all your nutrients in one meal and call it a day. But that's like expecting a magic trick from a nun—sometimes, life doesn't work that way. Instead, aim for a balanced diet throughout the day. Don't worry if you can't have the world's most perfect meal in one sitting.

Let's say you start with a breakfast that includes bread, eggs, fruit, and maybe a vegetable, and wash it down with fruit juice or water. That's a solid start, right? If that's too much, no problem! Have some calorie-dense bread and eggs now, and a nutrient-packed salad later. Get creative, like a mad scientist mixing up healthy concoctions. Your body will thank you later (probably).

So, eat your carbs, proteins, fats, and vitamins like you're assembling a superhero team. Make sure each one has its role, and try to avoid the temptation of just loading up on cake, at least until after lunch.

4.4.6.   Health Benefits of a Balanced Diet

Improved Physical Health: Let's face it: your body needs food to survive, but not just any food. You need the good stuff—carbs, proteins, and all those vitamins that sound too boring to care about but do wonders like keeping your cells from disintegrating after that catastrophic fall down the stairs. A balanced diet gives your body the tools to perform miracles, like healing itself, growing, and fighting off all those nasty illnesses that love to pop up out of nowhere.

Eat well, and you can lower your risk of the big, scary diseases like cancer, heart disease, stroke, and T2DM, which are basically the body's way of sending a message: *"Hey, you really should've eaten that salad."* Plus, your waistline will thank you as you keep that "healthy weight" tag in check, leaving you with more energy to avoid the zombie-like state of exhaustion we all know too well.

Mental Health Benefits: Believe it or not, what you shove into your mouth can affect your mood. So, if you're feeling like an emotional wreck, maybe it's time to ditch the junk food and try some whole grains, veggies, and lean protein. These nutrient-packed foods can calm your brain, reduce stress, and, if you're lucky, stop you from calling your ex at 2 a.m. Studies even suggest that a balanced diet can help you fight off depression and anxiety like a mental superhero, improving brain function, and making you less likely to cry in public.

Increased Energy Levels: If you're constantly yawning, running on fumes, and wondering how you can possibly make it through the day without face-planting into your desk, your diet might be to blame. A balanced diet, with a steady dose of complex carbs and lean protein, can keep your energy levels from plunging into the abyss. No more mid-afternoon crashes—just pure, unadulterated productivity (or at least the ability to keep your eyes open without drooling). Plus, a healthy diet can help you sleep better so you can get through tomorrow without trying to navigate life on autopilot.

Improved Digestion: Digestive problems? Oh, the horror. Nobody wants to spend their day feeling bloated, constipated, or wondering why their stomach is throwing a tantrum. A balanced diet, full of fibre-rich foods, ensures that everything moves through your digestive system like a well-oiled machine. You'll be regular, so you can leave your bathroom anxieties behind and focus on more important things, like binge-watching your favourite show without interruption.

Better Skin Health: Want to look younger, more radiant, and like you actually slept? A balanced diet rich in vitamins, minerals, and antioxidants can help banish acne, wrinkles, and other skin issues that seem to multiply the moment you hit adulthood. Say goodbye to looking like you've been hit with a bad case of the flu, and hello to glowing skin that makes you look like you have your life together (even if you don't).

Improved Immune System: You know those days when you feel like the walking dead because you caught every bug going around? Well, a balanced diet, full of essential nutrients, can keep your immune system in tip-top shape, so you're less likely to catch that cold that's been circulating for the past three months. Goodbye, sniffles. Hello, health!

Support Antioxidant Function: Antioxidants are your body's bouncers, keeping free radicals from causing chaos and prematurely aging you. Fruits and veggies are your go-to for a solid supply of these bad boys, so start munching on them like your life depends on it—because, let's be honest, it kinda does.

Maintain Gut Health: Your gut's like a petting zoo—full of microorganisms doing their best to keep you healthy. Give them the right food, and they'll keep you strong. A diet full of fibre-rich foods is the VIP pass to a happy gut, meaning better digestion and, hopefully, fewer awkward stomach growls in public.

Reduce Inflammation: Chronic inflammation is basically your immune system throwing a tantrum, and guess what? A balanced diet can calm it down. Anti-inflammatory foods like nuts, seeds, and fatty fish work wonders to keep things chill so your immune system doesn't go into full meltdown mode at the slightest inconvenience.

Promote a Healthy Body Weight: Carrying around extra weight isn't just a fashion problem—it can mess with your immune system and make it harder to fight off infections. A balanced diet can help keep your weight in check, reduce calorie intake, and provide the proper nutrients to ensure your body stays in fighting shape. Because, let's face it, the only thing you should be fighting is your craving for that fifth slice of pizza.

A balanced diet isn't just about looking good—though that's a nice bonus—it's about making sure you're functioning properly, from your immune system to your brain. Eating right will give you the edge, whether it's better skin, improved energy, or finally beating the digestive demons. So, put down that donut and pick up that apple (unless it's in a pie—then we'll talk).

5. Gaining Weight

If you consume more calories than your body needs or burn fewer calories than you consume, congratulations—you've cracked the code for gaining weight! Your body, ever the efficient hoarder, will lovingly store the excess as fat, just in case you ever decide to take up hibernation. This magic number of calories your body needs to keep you alive and functioning is called your Daily Energy Expenditure (DEE). Think of it as your personal calorie budget. Spend wisely, or your body will turn into a storage unit for extra energy.

Factors like your age, gender, weight, height, and how often you pretend to enjoy exercise determine your DEE. Go over this number, and your body will dutifully pack on the pounds. It's like your metabolism saying, *"Oh, you're not burning this? Cool, I'll save it for later."*

Then, there's the glorious option of physical inactivity. Skip the gym, embrace the couch, and let YouTube autoplay your life into a sedentary blur. Whether by cutting down on workouts or doubling down on naps, reducing your activity level ensures your body will gleefully convert all those extra calories into fat. You're basically a human battery, storing energy for a rainy day that never comes.

5.1. Consuming More Calories

The key to maintaining a healthy weight is simple: balance calorie intake and energy expenditure. Easier said than done, of course, because your body treats excess calories like a squirrel hoarding nuts for winter—except there's no winter, just tighter jeans and existential regret.

Skipping meals might seem like a shortcut to weight loss, but it's really just a booby trap set by your own appetite. Sure, you might feel like a hunger warrior at first, but give it a few hours, and your stomach will turn into a demanding toddler, screaming for high-calorie foods. Eventually, you'll cave and inhale an entire pizza, effectively turning your earlier fasting into a calorie bomb. Well played, body.

Here's another fun scenario: You start your day with a heroic 3,000-calorie breakfast, thinking it'll carry you through. Spoiler alert: by noon, your stomach is already auditioning for a horror movie with those growls. By evening, if you haven't eaten, you'll probably devour another 3,000 calories to appease your angry belly, except this time, you won't have the time to burn those evening calories—your body's just tucking them away for its fat collection. It's like a very unprofitable investment portfolio.

Not tracking calorie intake is like driving a car with no speedometer—you might be fine, or you might crash into a double cheeseburger at 160 km/h or 100 mph. You don't have to obsessively count every calorie like it's your retirement fund, but maybe consider knowing if your snack is the equivalent of a light jog or a marathon with an Ethiopian Olympian. The bottom line? Be mindful of what you eat because every bite counts—literally, on the scale.

5.2. Using Fewer Calories

Reducing physical activity is like inviting weight gain to crash on your couch—and trust me, it's not leaving anytime soon. A sedentary lifestyle means your body burns calories at the pace of a sloth napping under a palm tree. Combine that with an extra snack (or five), and you're essentially running a weight-gain charity.

When you're physically inactive, your body becomes the ultimate minimalist: it doesn't expend energy unless absolutely necessary. So, while you're binge-watching your favourite crime drama marathon, your body is busy storing all those extra calories like a bear preparing for winter—except the bear in you never hibernates and stores food all year round.

Even simple movements like housework or walking are calorie-burning heroes. But spend too much time glued to your desk chair, and your metabolism will slow down like it's on strike. Fun fact: sitting burns so few calories that if laziness ever becomes a sport, it will be the most popular Olympic sport. The only sport where participants can be viewers and vice versa.

The moral of the story? If you want to avoid turning into a human beanbag, get up, move around, and remind your body that it's not just a fat storage unit.

5.3. Common Behaviours

Turns out, gaining weight is easier than finding matching socks in the morning. Everyday habits—those sneaky little routines—are often the culprits behind our expanding waistlines. But don't worry, understanding these habits isn't rocket science (although it might feel like it after a midnight snack binge). Let's dive in and unravel the mystery of why your jeans are conspiring against you—and maybe, just maybe, make some healthier choices along the way.

5.3.1. Overeating

Overeating: the art of turning a casual meal into a competitive sport. Whether it's that one glorious buffet sitting or snacking your way through the day like a human vacuum, your body takes every extra calorie and whispers, *"Don't worry, I'll save this for later!"* Spoiler alert: "for later" means in your thighs.

Here's the math nobody asked for: 3,500 extra calories = 1 pound of 'fun.' You can rack that up in one sitting (hello, family-sized pizza for yours truly, only) or spread it out over weeks of innocent "just one more bite" moments. Either way, the calories don't care—they're just here to crash on your couch...forever.

5.3.2.   Excess Calorie-Dense Foods

High-calorie foods: where the taste buds party, and your waistline gets the hangover. Enter the stars of the show: processed snacks and sugary drinks, the edible equivalent of gas station lottery tickets—lots of excitement, zero payoffs.

Take a can of pop, for instance. At 200 calories a pop (pun intended), you might think, *"What harm could one do?"* The answer? Plenty. Because minutes later, you're staring at an empty can, still hungry, and the siren call of the next can is impossible to ignore. Before you know it, you've hit your DEE in sugar-water, and regret was the only thing it gave back.

Fun fact: these "empty calories" are so **nutrient-deficient** that they make your body beg for more food to compensate. And what do you give it? Another pop. Congratulations, you've just turned your stomach into a vending machine—except this one only dispenses disappointment and spare tires around your waist.

5.3.3.   Lack of Physical Activity

Physical activity is that thing we all swear we'll start next week but somehow ends up on next year's to-do list. Regular movement keeps your calorie-burning engine revved up, preventing your body from turning into a long-term storage unit for unused snacks.

When you're active, your muscles bulk up like eager employees at a metabolism factory, burning calories even while you binge-watch TV with one hand down your pants. But skip leg day—or all the days—and those muscles will peace out faster than a bad Hinge date. This muscle shrinkage, also known as muscle atrophy, is your body's way of saying, "If you're not gonna use it, I'm not gonna keep it." Yes, you'd have become "unhinged" (get it?).

The result? DEE takes a nosedive (pun intended), but your eating habits? Still living large. And that's how you end up starring in your own personal episode of "When Calories Attack." Moral of the story: move it, or lose it… and then gain it back in the form of fat.

5.3.4.   Poor Food Choices

Unhealthy food choices are like the toxic ex that keeps sliding into DMs, disguised as a comforting late-night snack (pun intended). Processed, high-fat foods are the attention-seeking celebrities of the food world: calorie-dense, attention-grabbing, and everywhere you turn.

Here's the math of your misery: every gram of fat is like a nine-calorie time bomb waiting to explode in your body. Meanwhile, carbs are the underachievers, needing twice the effort to deliver the same nine calories. Carbs only carry four calories per gram. So, when you opt for that double cheeseburger, you're basically taking the express lane to caloric overload with a side of regret.

Let's not forget inflammation—the party crasher of your internal systems. It shows up uninvited, bringing chronic diseases like obesity, T2DM, and heart disease to the festivities. Bottom line: choosing calorie-dense foods is like playing Russian roulette with your health… you never know which bullet made of extra butter will take you out (pun intended).

5.3.5.   Lack of Sleep

Sleep, everyone's favourite free therapy session. But here's the thing: if you're not getting enough of it, your body will start messing with you like a bad ex. Lack of sleep throws your hormones into a frenzy, particularly the ones that tell you when you're hungry and when you're full. Suddenly, you find yourself craving junk food at 2 a.m., like your body is pleading with you to sabotage your diet.

Your **circadian rhythms**—the biological equivalent of a grandmaster clock—control this chaos. These rhythms run on a 24-hour cycle, keeping your body in sync with the environment. When it's dark, melatonin, your sleep hormone, says *"goodnight."*

But when it's morning, cortisol comes out to play, making sure you're wide awake and ready to conquer the world.

Now, if you're a night owl, this is where things get ugly. Your body is literally programmed to sleep when it's dark and eat during the day, but night shifts throw that system into chaos. You're awake when your metabolism is sluggish and asleep when it's working its hardest, making weight gain inevitable. So, in a nutshell, **sleep deprivation** isn't just making you grumpy—it's turning you into a calorie-hoarding machine.

5.3.6. Stress Eating

Who needs emotional stability when you can have an entire pint of ice cream instead? When life throws its curveballs, many of us instinctively turn to food for comfort. Unfortunately, food doesn't exactly return the favour with a "there, there" hug. Instead, it piles on the calories, often in the form of unhealthy, high-calorie junk that's just begging for your emotional breakdown.

And then there's cortisol, the 'stress hormone' that pops up like an unwanted guest at the party. Cortisol's main job is to make you crave more food, ensuring that the stress-induced snack fest doesn't end anytime soon. While a bit of acute stress might actually speed up your metabolism—because, hey, we all need that adrenaline rush—chronic stress is a whole different ball game. It messes with your ability to burn fat, leaving your body perfectly content to store all those extra calories. So, congrats! Not only are you stressed, but you're also putting on the pounds in the process.

5.3.7. Skipping Meals

Apparently, starving yourself is a "genius" weight loss strategy, right? Well, not quite. When you skip a meal, your body thinks it's about to enter a famine apocalypse, so it slows your metabolism to conserve energy. And when you finally decide to eat, your body holds on to every last calorie, just in case you try to starve it again. This may come off as mean-spirited, but this is nature's genius way of keeping you alive in the event of another period of starvation.

But that's not the only issue. Missing a meal doesn't just mean saving calories— you're setting yourself up for an all-you-can-eat buffet later. Skipping meals leaves you feeling deprived, which naturally leads to overcompensating with larger portions or, let's be real, a mountain of junk food. Suddenly, your "sensible" calorie deficit is looking more like a calorie avalanche.

Let's not forget about hormones—the real drama queens of weight management. Skipping breakfast, for example, sends leptin (your body's 'chill, you're full' signal) into hiding and sends ghrelin (the 'I'm starving, feed me everything' hormone) into overdrive. This hormonal cocktail of hunger chaos ensures that you'll be eating more than you ever intended—and with a side of guilt, naturally.

5.3.8.   Alcohol Consumption

This magical liquid that helps you forget your problems for only a couple of hours also adds to your waistline in a way that makes your one-size-fits-all stretch pants blush. Let's break it down: a pint of beer? 150 calories. A glass of wine? Same thing. A shot of vodka or whiskey? Only 100 calories—just enough to make you feel tipsy but not tipsy enough to forget about that muffin top. Think about it: a six-pack of beer is like consuming 900 calories of regret, a bottle of wine is 700 calories of *"I should've found a better way to deal with life,"* and five shots of whiskey are about 500 calories of *"I'll just have one more, what's the worst that could happen?"*

But wait, there's more! Alcohol doesn't just sit there in your stomach like a good little drink. Oh no, it actively sabotages your metabolism, slowing it down like a Tesla with a dying battery. Instead of burning fat, your body is too busy trying to process the booze, storing that fat like it's a Thursday before Black Friday, and it's got to stock up. Nice, right?

If you think alcohol is just making you fat in a silent, sneaky way, think again. It also messes with your decision-making. One drink turns into five, and suddenly, you're eating an extra-large pizza with extra cheese by yourself at 3 a.m. with a gallon of pop to wash it down because your judgment's gone the way of your dignity. Plus, those sugary cocktails? They'll make you crave all the wrong foods, like your ex's phone number... and more pizza.

As if that wasn't enough, alcohol decides to ruin your sleep, too. It knocks you out, but doesn't let you truly rest, which means your hunger hormones are running wild the next day. Dehydration from drinking? Oh, that's just the cherry on top, leading to even worse decision-making and a metabolism that's like, *"Nope, I'm on vacation."* Cheers to that, right?

5.4. Less Common Behaviours

In addition to the everyday habits that can lead to weight gain, some lesser-known lifestyle habits can sneak up on you like a surprise pizza delivery. Let's dive in, shall we?

5.4.1. Medications

Medications are meant to help, but sometimes they're like that one friend who shows up to your party uninvited with his grandmother and "new girlfriend's" infant because he couldn't find a sitter for them. If you've noticed your waistband tightening, it might not just be your love of nachos—it could be those pills you're popping. Here's a rundown of common culprits:

5.4.1.1. Antidepressants (SSRIs and SNRIs)

They're supposed to make you feel better mentally but might worsen your waistline. Some antidepressants can increase appetite or slow your metabolism. So, while you're trying to feel happy, your body is over here saying, *"You know what would make you even happier? A pint of ice cream."* Thanks, meds.

5.4.1.2. Antipsychotics

These meds are often prescribed to manage conditions like schizophrenia or bipolar disorder. Unfortunately, they can also mess with your body's hormones and appetite regulation. The result? A sudden, uninvited increase in hunger and a decrease in metabolism. Think of it like a party in your stomach where only high-calorie foods are allowed.

5.4.1.3.   Corticosteroids (like Prednisone)

These little pills are powerful for treating inflammation and autoimmune diseases, but they can also cause **fluid retention** and an increase in hunger. So, while you're treating your condition, you might also end up with some extra baggage (literally). Your body's like, *"I'm swollen with joy, and it's sticking around!"*

5.4.1.4.   Diabetes Medications (Insulin and Sulfonylureas)

While these meds are crucial for managing blood sugar levels, they can also cause weight gain. Insulin helps your body store glucose, and sometimes that means storing a little extra fat along with it. And sulfonylureas increase insulin production, which can have the same effect on your waistline. It's like your body gets the message to store fat, and it takes it very seriously.

5.4.1.5.   Beta-Blockers

Prescribed for heart conditions like slowing your heart rate to lower your blood pressure, beta-blockers can also slow your metabolism and reduce your ability to burn fat efficiently. So, while you're keeping your heart healthy, your body might just be chilling in fat storage mode. It's the ultimate "slow and steady" approach to weight gain.

5.4.1.6.   Antihistamines

These allergy meds are great for stopping you from sneezing, but they might also increase your appetite or decrease your metabolic rate. So, while you're breathing easy, your pants might be getting a little tighter.

5.4.1.7.   Mood Stabilizers (like Lithium)

Used to treat bipolar disorder, lithium can lead to weight gain through mechanisms like fluid retention, changes in metabolism, and increased hunger. It's like your body gets a message that it should keep everything—including extra calories—on hand for "just in case."

5.4.1.8.   Hormone Replacement Therapy (HRT)

HRT the lifeline for some during the transition through perimenopause and beyond—can also be a culprit in the battle of the bulge. While it's designed to replace the estrogen your body no longer produces, that estrogen can sometimes get a bit too comfortable and decide to store a little extra fat. The hormonal shift can increase insulin resistance, making your body more likely to stash fat—especially around your hips and thighs. And let's not forget the lovely side effect of fluid retention, turning you into a walking water balloon. Not precisely the glow-up you were hoping for, huh?

5.4.1.9.   Oral Contraceptive Pills (OCPs)

OCPs are often hailed as convenient and reliable, but they can come with a side order of weight gain. They are packed with progesterone, a hormone that has a not-so-friendly effect on your appetite. You know those days before your period when you can eat an entire pizza and still crave chocolate? Yeah, that's progesterone working its magic. Progesterone stimulates the hunger centres in your brain, which can leave you raiding the fridge at 2 a.m. So, while OCPs are great at preventing pregnancy, they're also really good at promoting a serious snack attack.

If your body isn't eliminating these meds properly (say, through hydration and fibre), the accumulation of progesterone can lead to a toxic overload. The symptoms? Oh, just some lovely PMS-like effects: bloating, breast tenderness, mood swings, irritability, and, of course, weight gain. It's like your body gets the worst part of your cycle without even needing to check the calendar.

It's important to note that not everyone who takes HRT or OCPs will gain weight, and if you do, it may not be a drastic change. But if you notice the pounds creeping up, talk to your healthcare provider. They can adjust your dosage or suggest alternatives so you can get the benefits of the meds without the unwanted "extra luggage." After all, the only thing that should be increasing is your happiness—not your waistline.

5.4.2. Hormonal Imbalances

Hormones are like the unsung managers of your body, directing everything from metabolism to hunger. But when they get out of whack, it's like your body starts throwing a tantrum and decides to pile on the pounds.

Take insulin, for instance. Insulin's job is to regulate blood sugar levels and help your body store fat. But if your insulin levels stay high—whether due to insulin resistance or other factors—your body thinks, *"Hey, let's just keep storing fat, no big deal,"* and you end up gaining weight. It's like your body has a pantry that never stops filling up, but never gets around to using any food inside.

Then there's the thyroid, that little butterfly-shaped gland at the base of your neck. Thyroid hormones (T3 and T4) are in charge of regulating your metabolism. If you've got an underactive thyroid (hypothyroidism), your metabolism goes into snooze mode, and weight gain is the unwelcome side effect. On the flip side, an overactive thyroid (hyperthyroidism) can send your metabolism into overdrive, leading to weight loss. It's a hormonal game of Goldilocks—too slow or too fast, but never just right.

Estrogen and progesterone, those two hormone heavyweights, also throw their weight around, particularly when it comes to women's bodies. Estrogen helps with fertility and menstrual cycles, but too much or too little of it can cause weight gain, especially during perimenopause or after menopause. Meanwhile, progesterone is like that friend who can't stop offering you snacks. When your progesterone levels spike (right before your period), it signals your brain to go full hunger mode, which explains why you feel like you could eat an entire pizza just before Aunt Flo arrives.

And don't forget about cortisol, the stress hormone. We've talked about how it can cause weight gain when your body's in fight-or-flight mode, but when cortisol is chronically elevated, it can prompt your body to hang onto fat like a security blanket. It's like your body thinks it's under constant threat of some giant, stress-inducing monster, so it holds on to fat just in case.

Of course, everyone's hormones are unique, and weight gain can come from a complex cocktail of factors. But if your hormones aren't in harmony, you might find yourself packing on the pounds without even realizing why.

5.4.3. Poor Gut Health

Your gut microbiome is like the unruly roommates you never asked for. It lives in your digestive tract and decides how everything operates—whether it's your metabolism, digestion, or weight. When these bacteria get out of balance, a condition known as **gut dysbiosis**, it's like a party gone wrong, and your body is left to deal with the consequences.

For one, an unhealthy gut can spark inflammation, making it harder for your body to properly absorb nutrients from your food. This can cause **nutritional deficiencies**, which makes your body think it's starving, so it ramps up hunger. Your stomach's like, *"Feed me more!"* leading to overeating and—surprise!—weight gain.

Gut bacteria also play a role in controlling hunger and fullness through hormones like ghrelin and leptin. When your gut bacteria are off-kilter, you might see ghrelin levels rise, cranking up your appetite, while leptin levels drop, signalling to your brain that you're still hungry, even when you're not. Essentially, it's like your body's hunger signals get all mixed up, causing you to raid the fridge and pantry and pack on the pounds.

And let's not forget about glucose metabolism. When your gut bacteria are out of whack, they mess with your body's ability to absorb glucose and regulate insulin. This can lead to insulin resistance, a metabolic issue that's often linked to weight gain. It's like your body's insulin is knocking on the door to use the sugar, but no one's home to answer, so it just keeps storing fat instead.

Stress and a diet rich in sugar and processed foods don't help either. They can add more fuel to the fire, creating the perfect storm for a gut microbiome disaster. To keep everything in check, focus on a fibre-packed, probiotic, and prebiotic-rich diet, and remember to manage your stress. Treat your gut right, and it might just stop sabotaging your weight management efforts.

5.5. Common Medical Conditions

Certain medical conditions are like the sneaky troublemakers of the weight gain world, silently throwing off your body's metabolic processes or messing with the hormones that control weight. Here are a few of them, playing their parts in the never-ending battle with the scale:

5.5.1. Hypothyroidism

Hypothyroidism is like having a slow, underperforming engine in your body. Your thyroid, that little butterfly-shaped gland in your neck, just can't seem to get it together and produces too few thyroid hormones. These hormones are supposed to keep your metabolism revved up, but when they're slacking off, your metabolism hits the brakes. This means your body burns fewer calories, and suddenly, you're carrying around extra weight with little effort.

When metabolism takes a nosedive, your body becomes terrible at breaking down food, leading to fluid retention and hunger pangs that just won't quit. People with hypothyroidism often feel sluggish, like they've just woken up from a year-long nap, which leads to less movement and an even slower metabolic rate. It's like your body has decided to skip the gym and chill on the couch all day.

As if that weren't enough, hypothyroidism can change where your body stores fat. It's like your body has its own "fat redistribution plan," shifting weight to the abdomen and hips, making it harder to lose. And the worst part? Without treatment, this hormonal mess continues, and losing that weight is like trying to shovel snow with a teaspoon—slow and almost impossible.

In short, hypothyroidism slows your metabolism and makes everything harder—losing weight, staying active, and feeling warm—a real package deal!

5.5.2. Polycystic Ovarian Syndrome (PCOS)

PCOS is a hormonal rollercoaster for women, and not the fun kind. It's a tangled mess of symptoms like irregular periods, infertility, excessive hair growth (hello, moustache), acne, and, of course, weight gain. This weight gain isn't just a byproduct; it's one of the most persistent and frustrating symptoms of PCOS, and it's all due to a few sneaky culprits.

Insulin Resistance: Many women with PCOS have insulin resistance, meaning their bodies struggle to use insulin effectively. As a result, insulin levels rise, and all that extra glucose just gets turned into fat. And where does this fat love to settle? Of course, the abdominal area makes it even harder to shake off.

Hormonal Imbalance: In addition to insulin problems, PCOS causes an overload of androgens, which are the "male hormones" women don't need (but unfortunately get). These hormones play a sneaky role in increasing belly fat. And, because they mess with how your body processes insulin, they make weight gain even more inevitable. Great.

Inflammation: PCOS is often accompanied by low-grade inflammation, which amps up the production of cytokines. These little guys aren't your friends—they encourage your body to store more fat, particularly around the midsection. It's like inflammation has something personal it is trying to get back to you about.

Lack of Physical Activity: Fatigue is a common issue with PCOS, and when you're exhausted all the time, hitting the gym feels like an impossible task. Less exercise means more weight gain, which causes even more fatigue, and before you know it, you're stuck in an endless cycle.

But there's hope! Losing weight with PCOS may be tough, but it's not impossible. Managing the condition through a healthy diet (low in refined carbs, high in fibre), regular exercise, and medications to balance reproductive hormones and insulin can work wonders. In fact, weight loss can even help with other PCOS symptoms like irregular periods and fertility, making it a win-win for overall health.

5.5.3. Cushing's Syndrome

Cushing's syndrome is like your body throwing a non-stop party with cortisol, the stress hormone. Usually, cortisol helps regulate your metabolism, but when your body produces too much of it, it's like the metabolism becomes moody. High cortisol levels can lead to weight gain and a whole host of other symptoms. Here's how it all goes down:

Increased Appetite: Cortisol can trigger your hunger, making you crave food constantly. But it's not just any food—it's the kind that leads to weight gain, particularly in your belly. So, while you're battling cravings, your waistline is expanding, and your risk of issues like T2DM and heart disease is going up, too. Fun.

Fat Distribution: When cortisol goes rogue, it doesn't just deposit fat anywhere—it targets your belly. This "central obesity" is the kind of fat that's more likely to lead to health complications, making it not only frustrating but also dangerous.

Decreased Muscle Mass: Cortisol doesn't stop at increasing fat; it also breaks down muscle. This means less muscle mass, and your body burns fewer calories with less muscle. And guess what happens next? More weight gain. It's a vicious cycle where you can't lose weight as easily because muscle burns calories like a furnace, but now you're stuck with less of it.

Impaired Glucose Tolerance: Cortisol loves to mess with insulin, which is supposed to help your body use glucose for energy. But with cortisol throwing a wrench in the works, your cells become less responsive to insulin, leading to insulin resistance. This makes fat cells extra eager to store sugar as fat, and guess what? More weight gain.

Weight gain from Cushing's syndrome is tricky to reverse, but it's not impossible. The key is treating the root cause: lowering cortisol levels. Depending on the severity, this may involve medications to suppress cortisol production, surgery to remove the adrenal gland or any tumours, or even radiation therapy. On top of that, lifestyle changes—like exercise and a healthy diet—can help manage the symptoms and promote some weight loss. It might be a tough road, but it's not one you have to walk alone.

5.5.4. Sleep Disorders

Sleep is that thing we all pretend to get enough of while secretly binge-watching TV dramas until 3 a.m. Well, surprise! Lack of sleep isn't just going to leave you looking like a zombie; it might actually make you one—of the snack-eating variety. When you don't get enough shut-eye, your body throws a temper tantrum, releasing hormones that turn you into a hungry monster with cravings for high-calorie foods. Suddenly, your salad looks like a cruel joke, and that half-empty pizza box? Well, that's practically a health food.

Chronic sleep deprivation also messes with your metabolism. It's like your body's internal thermostat just gave up. Your metabolism slows down, and your body says, *"Hey, let's just store all this food for later... just in case we run into a famine or a bad reality TV show marathon."*

So, if you want to avoid looking like a hibernating bear who's gotten way too comfy on the couch, try actually sleeping. It's not just for your sanity; it might help you keep from turning into a walking snack cabinet.

5.6. Less Common Medical Conditions

Here are some less common medical conditions that can lead to weight gain:

5.6.1. Genetic Disorders

The gift that keeps on giving. Sometimes, it's not just your parents' questionable fashion choices that you inherit; it's also the charming ability to gain weight at the slightest hint of food. Here are some genetic conditions that don't just mess with your metabolism—they turn it into a full-on circus act:

5.6.1.1. Prader-Willi Syndrome

Imagine if your body thought "never-ending buffet" was a reasonable lifestyle. That's what Prader-Willi syndrome does to you. It's like your brain's "I'm full!" signal was lost in the mail, leaving you with an appetite that could rival a bottomless pit. Thanks to a malfunctioning hypothalamus and a growth hormone deficiency, it's like your stomach's Wi-Fi is permanently connected to an all-you-can-eat buffet.

5.6.1.2. Bardet-Biedl Syndrome

If your body were a dysfunctional tech startup, Bardet-Biedl syndrome would be the glitchy CEO. This rare genetic disorder messes with your appetite and gives your metabolism the middle finger. The mechanics of how it works are still a mystery, but it's like your hormones—especially leptin and insulin—decided to call in sick, and you're left hungry and stuck in a body that refuses to lose weight.

5.6.1.3. Alström Syndrome

Ever wonder what would happen if someone tried to make a hybrid between a human and a potato? Welcome to Alström syndrome! This delightful condition impacts your organs and systems like your eyes, heart, and liver, but it also brings the gift of insatiable hunger. Think of it as your body being in a constant "snack attack" mode, with a side of weight gain. It's like your brain just can't find the "I'm full" button, and it will never stop trying to eat everything in sight.

5.6.1.4. Leptin Deficiency

Leptin is the body's little voice of reason, saying, *"Hey, maybe stop eating that fourth serving of pizza."* But if you're lucky enough to have a genetic deficiency in leptin, your body misses that memo entirely. You end up with a stomach that's basically a bottomless pit while your brain just sits there, blissfully unaware that it's supposed to be telling you to stop shovelling food into your face.

In some cases, some medications or therapies might help dial down the madness. But don't get too excited—it's a case-by-case, *"let's see if we can at least make things a little less catastrophic"* approach. So, if you find yourself gaining weight faster than your social media feed updates, maybe it's time to consider that genetics might have thrown in a little too much help. However, these genetic conditions are so rare that less than 1% of 1% are likely affected. Also, if you blew up after you started first grade, it's unlikely that it's one of these gifts from Mother Nature making you banned from every buffet in town.

5.6.2. Imbalance of Reproductive Hormones

Hormonal imbalances, like low testosterone and estrogen, are another way human biology gives you the middle finger when it comes to weight management. Here's how they do it:

5.6.2.1.　Low Testosterone

Testosterone is basically the body's personal trainer. When it's on vacation, your metabolism takes a nap, and your muscles decide to leave the party. The result? You're stuck with more fat, especially in the dreaded belly area. So now, even if you try your best to diet and exercise, your body's just like, *"Yeah, we're good with this extra weight, thanks."*

But wait, there's more! Low testosterone doesn't just want to make your abs disappear; it also takes your energy levels down with it. Testosterone boosts your energy by making more red blood cells and getting glucose to do its job. When that's low, it's like someone turned off the lights, and suddenly, your workout is just a distant dream. Low energy? More fat. It's like your body is plotting against you.

5.6.2.2.　Low Estrogen

Estrogen, the hormone that helps women stay lean and mean, apparently thinks dropping the ball as you age is funny. When estrogen goes on strike, your body's metabolism turns into a sluggish sloth, and fat—especially around the belly—decides to set up camp. So, while your body desperately tries to burn calories, estrogen is over there snacking on chips, chilling in the corner, and watching your fat stores increase.

Estrogen also messes with how your body distributes fat. It's like the lousy roommate who rearranges your furniture for fun—only it's your fat, and it's moved into the most inconvenient areas. The abdomen becomes a VIP section for extra pounds, making weight loss feel like a cruel joke.

Hormonal imbalances can be caused by everything from getting older to having genes that seem to hate you. Treating them usually involves a mix of meds, hormone therapy, or pretending to enjoy broccoli and exercise. But don't worry, as long as your hormones are out of whack, there's always an excuse for why you can't fit into those skinny jeans.

5.6.3.   Chronic Stress

Chronic stress is like that toxic friend who keeps showing up uninvited, bringing all kinds of chaos—including hormonal imbalances and weight gain. Let's dive into the hormonal mess that stress creates:

5.6.3.1.   Cortisol

The hormone that floods your system when your boss asks you for that last-minute report or your internet cuts out right before a deadline. This hormone, produced by your adrenal glands, is your body's version of "fight or flight," or, more realistically, "eat an entire pizza because life's not fair." When cortisol levels stay elevated from chronic stress, it's like your body's emergency system is permanently stuck in overdrive.

Cortisol tells your liver to release glycogen (aka stored sugar) into your bloodstream. Great for fighting off that sabretooth tiger, but not so much for dealing with the stress of finding your car keys. The problem? If cortisol sticks around too long, you develop insulin resistance. Basically, your body's like, *"Yeah, we don't need that glucose right now"* (except fat cells—fat cells are still down for the snack party). So, your fat cells happily store all the glucose your body can't use. You're not using it, but your body's sure as hell saving it.

5.6.3.2.   Insulin

The hormone that's supposed to keep your blood sugar levels in check. Stress also throws a wrench into insulin's work, causing it to become less effective. So, while your body still has cortisol hanging around like an unwanted guest at a party, insulin gets lazy and doesn't bother storing sugar properly. Instead, that sugar gets packed away as fat because, why not? Your body's clearly decided that fat is the new black.

5.6.3.3.　Appetite

Stress isn't content just messing with your metabolism—it's also here to wreck your appetite. Chronic stress cranks up your hunger hormone, ghrelin, and knocks down leptin, the one that tells you when you're full. So, you end up in a vicious cycle of being constantly hungry and craving all the unhealthy, high-calorie foods that your body so desperately needs... to deal with stress. It's like your body's saying, *"You can't handle life? Fine, here's an entire box of donuts."* Stress eating isn't just about emotional comfort; it's your body throwing a tantrum and demanding food to cope with the chaos it's created.

To avoid becoming a stress-fuelled snack monster, managing stress with some sanity-saving habits, like exercise, mindfulness, or even hiding in a closet for five minutes of peace, is crucial. And don't forget about diet, sleep, and some good ol' "physical activity"—they'll help get your hormones in check so you're not fighting off a muffin top just to fit into the little black dress you got for Christmas.

5.6.4.　Alcohol Consumption

Everyone's favourite liquid diet sabotage. Let's explore how it fattens your wallet and your waistline.

5.6.4.1.　Calorie Bomb

First, let's talk calories. Alcohol is like that sneaky friend who shows up uninvited to the party—except it brings seven calories per gram, just shy of fat's 9 per gram. So, when you down that 6-pack or bottle of wine, it's basically like inviting a thousand empty calories to your body's all-you-can-eat buffet. And what does alcohol do when it enters your system? It doesn't just sit there quietly—it stirs up a hunger for junk food that your body doesn't even need. But hey, who can resist those nachos when you're three margaritas deep?

5.6.4.2.　Metabolic Mayhem

Next up, alcohol's favourite party trick: it totally wrecks your metabolism. Your liver, which usually handles all the fat-burning responsibilities like a well-oiled machine, is now too busy processing alcohol. It's like your liver got a ticket to an all-you-can-drink bar and forgot it had a job the next morning. Meanwhile, your blood sugar's like, *"Hey, wait a minute!"* and starts hoarding sugar because it can't get the memo that it should process it. This leaves you with a nice little gift: insulin resistance, fat accumulation in your liver, and a body that's like, *"More alcohol, please!"* Which, surprise, surprise, leads to weight gain.

5.6.4.3. Appetite Awakening

Oh, but the fun doesn't stop there. Alcohol triggers your appetite like a switch. Your body's like, *"Oh great, I can't burn fat or sugar, but you know what sounds good? More food!"* And not just any food—nope. It craves high-calorie, high-fat delights. Thanks to the metabolic disaster happening inside, your body's pretty much screaming, *"Feed me, Seymour!"* while you're eyeing that pizza. On top of that, alcohol makes it so you don't want to move too much—coordination goes out the window, and suddenly you're on the couch, half-eaten pizza in hand, while your body's like, *"We're burning no calories today, pal."*

5.6.4.4. Fat Oxidation? More Like Fat Accumulation

If you were hoping alcohol would somehow help burn fat... surprise! It's actually more of a fat hoarder. While a little bit of sugar is burning away like a good little carb, alcohol prevents your body from burning fat for energy. So, instead of burning fat, your liver decides to pile it up like it's Black Friday and every fat cell is on sale. The sad thing is no one is buying. Fat in your blood? Yep. Fat in your liver? Absolutely. Fat in your tissue? You betcha. All that lovely fat will now hang out with the rest of your weight gain. Cheers!

5.6.4.5. Hormonal Havoc

Let's top it all off with hormones. Oh, alcohol, you're a hormonal troublemaker. Drinking too much booze can spike cortisol (aka the stress hormone), which is basically your body's invitation to pack on abdominal fat like it's a cozy winter coat. It also messes with hunger-regulating hormones, making you feel like you've never seen food before. And just to ensure the hormone chaos, chronic alcohol consumption can also mess with testosterone levels in men—yep, lower testosterone and higher estrogen. So, in short: hello belly fat, and good luck seeing your feet, maybe ever!

While alcohol might seem like your bestie for a night out, it's more like that friend who eats all the snacks and never does the dishes. If you want to keep your waistline in check and your liver from staging a revolt, it's probably a good idea to cut back on the booze. The American Heart Association recommends no more than two drinks a day for men and one for women (yes, even the human body is sexist). But hey, live your life—just remember that "beer belly" isn't just a catchy phrase; it's a life that chooses you if you're not careful.

5.6.5.   Aging

The joys of aging—when your body decides to start betraying you in all sorts of subtle ways, leading to weight gain. Let's break down how this delightful process unfolds:

5.6.5.1.   Decreased Metabolism

Remember when you could eat an entire pizza without gaining a pound? Yeah, those days are long gone. As you age, your metabolism slows down, and now your body burns fewer calories while you binge-watch Netflix or nap (let's be honest, that's 90% of your day). This slow-mo metabolism is partly due to your cells getting older and lazier—kind of like you, but on a microscopic level. Your heart also decides it's tired and drops a beat every year. And don't even get me started on your hormones, which are essentially throwing a pity party for themselves and can't be bothered to regulate hunger or metabolism properly anymore. Aging: the gift that keeps on giving.

5.6.5.2.   Decreased Muscle Mass

You're losing muscle, but hey, at least that means you don't have to carry around all that strength and energy, right? As you age, your muscle mass decreases because... well, you're not using it. If you don't use it, you lose it—and, much like your will to work out, it's gone. Fewer muscles mean fewer calories burned, which is essentially your body saying, *"Oh, you want to keep that weight off? Cute. Enjoy these extra pounds."* If you're still holding on to any semblance of dignity, resistance training is your best bet to keep muscle mass in check and avoid turning into a human marshmallow.

5.6.5.3.   Hormonal Changes

As you age, your hormone levels take a nosedive, like the excitement in your life after your 30s. Estrogen and testosterone, those delightful little buggers, start declining, and the next thing you know, your metabolism goes from a Ferrari to a tricycle. This results in more fat—particularly around your stomach—while your muscles quietly disappear. So, while your waistline expands, your once-toned body is asking you, *"What happened to the good old days?"*

5.6.5.4.   Medications

The pharmaceutical industry loves it when you age. Some of the medications you're now on, like antidepressants or steroids, can make weight gain their side gig. So, you get to enjoy all the joys of getting older, and now you also get to deal with the added bonus of your body packing on pounds like it's preparing for hibernation. Talk about a win-win, right?

5.6.5.5.   Poor Diet

Cooking a healthy meal? Ha! Who has the time or energy for that when you're knee-deep in processed foods and takeout menus? As you age, shopping for groceries or standing at the stove becomes more of a chore than a hobby. So, naturally, you rely on the convenient, calorie-packed foods that help maintain that nice, round figure. Your body thanks you by not letting go of those calories, even when you try to shake them off.

5.6.5.6. Inactivity and Sedentary Behaviour

At some point, moving becomes less of a priority and more of a *"do I really need to get up?"* kind of situation. Your joints start complaining every time you move, and the thought of being physically active becomes an exercise in mental gymnastics. Sitting around seems like a much better option, which is fantastic for YouTube but not so great for your waistline. But don't worry, if you can find something that doesn't hurt—like swimming—at least you'll be doing something good for your body, instead of just letting it grow into a human beanbag.

5.6.5.7. Chronic Stress

If aging wasn't stressful enough, now your body decides it's going to handle it all poorly. Chronic stress ramps up cortisol levels, which encourages your body to store fat—especially in the one place you don't want it: your stomach. So, while you're stressing over everything that's wrong with the world (or just the fact that your knees creak when you bend down), your body is like, *"Hey, let's just store this stress as belly fat."* Sounds like a fun time!

So, yeah, aging is excellent... if you're a fine wine. But if you're like most of us, the weight gain is just one more thing to deal with. To combat this delightful aging process, try maintaining a healthy diet (good luck), getting regular exercise (pain-free options preferred), and managing stress (because who isn't stressed about aging?). All of this will help you manage weight and maybe—just maybe—keep that muffin top from turning into a full-on cake.

5.6.6. Musculoskeletal problems

Here's how your achy joints and back pain are secretly plotting against you and your waistline:

5.6.6.1.   Decreased Physical Activity

When your body starts to protest against physical activity—thanks to joint pain, arthritis, or back issues—everything you used to love, like running, jumping, or even bending over to pick up the TV remote, becomes a battle. So, what's left? Sitting. Lots of sitting. And with sitting comes a decrease in your DEE, which basically means your body is just chilling while those calories sneak in. It's like your body's version of a lazy Sunday... every day. And the weight? It follows, like a clingy ex.

5.6.6.2.   Inactivity

Now, if you thought avoiding exercise was the answer, you're in for a treat. Musculoskeletal problems can make moving around a literal pain, which leads to more sitting or lying down. That's right; your body has now become a master in the fine art of sedentary living. The result? You burn fewer calories and pack on more weight while your joints (and your self-esteem) continue to deteriorate. It's a cycle of sitting, snacking, and sighing in discomfort.

5.6.6.3.   Chronic Pain

Chronic pain from musculoskeletal issues isn't just annoying; it's a mood killer. When you're in constant pain, stress, depression, and anxiety are your new roommates. What do these emotions love to do? Boost cortisol levels, which signals your body to store fat—particularly around your stomach. So, now, not only are you physically hurting, but your body decides to give you a little "bonus" belly fat to go along with it. Nothing says "fun" like stress-induced chub.

5.6.6.4.   Medications

When you finally cave in and take painkillers to numb the misery, you might find that the side effects come with their own problems. Some pain meds—especially opioids—don't just dull your pain; they also stimulate your appetite and slow down your metabolism.

So now you're eating more, burning fewer calories, and your body's like, *"Why not store some extra fat for later?"* Thanks, meds. You're a real pal.

5.6.6.5.   Reduced Range of Motion

If musculoskeletal issues weren't cruel enough, they also limit your ability to do exercises that can help you manage weight. For example, if you've got hip arthritis, performing simple movements like squats or lunges becomes more of a "please don't make me" situation. Without the full range of motion, you're essentially locked out of the fitness club, leaving you with fewer ways to keep those calories in check. It's like trying to play a video game with a broken controller.

So, what's a person with aching joints to do? Well, physical therapy, gentle exercises (like swimming or cycling—thankfully not too hard on the joints), and maybe even a healthy diet can help fight back. You know, the usual. But don't worry—your body will still find a way to remind you that it's getting older, one achy joint at a time.

6. Pregnancy

Pregnancy is the magical time when your body transforms into a 24/7 buffet for a tiny, demanding roommate who doesn't even pay rent. Sure, it's "special," but let's not sugarcoat it: the weight gain is inevitable, and while it's supposed to be "valuable," it also comes with its own set of "fun" complications.

First, let's get the warm and fuzzy part out of the way. Yes, weight gain during pregnancy is critical—it's how your body builds a cozy little habitat for the fetus, complete with all the essential nutrients, energy reserves, and, of course, a nice padding of fat to prep for breastfeeding. Think of it as your body stockpiling supplies for a nine-month marathon where you occasionally cry over spilled milk (literally) and lose your keys daily.

But let's not pretend this is all smooth sailing. The complications of pregnancy weight gain are like an exclusive version of regular weight-gain problems—bigger, worse, and now with bonus hormones. Swollen ankles, back pain, heartburn, and the delightful dance of trying to roll out of bed without resembling a turtle flipped on its shell. Plus, all those extra pounds don't just vanish post-baby; they linger, taunting you like an unwelcome guest at a party.

And don't get me started on the people who weigh in on your weight gain (pun absolutely intended). Your doctor tells you it's "normal," your husband says you're "glowing," and meanwhile, you're just trying to figure out if it's socially acceptable to eat an entire 2-pound cheesecake at 3 a.m. because the fetus demanded it.

So, yes, pregnancy weight gain is essential, but let's be honest— it's also a masterclass in how to navigate the line between necessary growth and feeling like a human beanbag. Hang in there, mom-to-be. At least your tiny tenant will eventually vacate... even if they leave the place a bit of a mess.

6.1. Gaining Weight During Pregnancy

6.1.1. Growing Baby

Let's start with the obvious: you're growing a tiny human. That little freeloading miracle requires energy, nutrients, and space, so your body transforms into a deluxe baby suite—complete with a bigger uterus and all the plush surroundings. Naturally, this adds to the scale, but hey, it's for a good cause. Your growing baby is the only time in life you'll gain weight and have people coo over it instead of giving you side-eye.

6.1.2. Fluid Retention

Fluid retention is the unsung villain of pregnancy weight gain. Your body starts producing more blood and fluids like it's stocking up for a drought. And while this sounds noble, it also means your ankles and feet might look like inflatable pool toys. Thanks to hydrostatic pressure (the force exerted on your blood vessels by the increased fluid), the increased fluid leaks into your tissues, forming edema—a fancy term for *"my feet look like marshmallows."* This fluid can't just disappear through your kidneys because, well, your body decided to keep it. So, congratulations, you're now waterlogged for nine months.

6.1.3. Hormonal Changes

Hormones are the puppet masters of your pregnancy, pulling all the strings to ensure you gain weight. Progesterone, for example, whispers sweet nothings to your metabolism, convincing it to slow down while simultaneously cranking up your appetite. And don't forget fat storage—your body's way of creating a snack pantry for labour and breastfeeding. Hormones essentially transform you into a walking Costco, stocked and ready for anything.

6.1.4. Food Intake

Finally, let's talk about food. Pregnancy is the only time society actively encourages you to eat more, and let's be honest, it's tempting to interpret "eating for two" as "eating two cheesecakes from Costco." Unfortunately, if those extra calories come from a steady diet of donuts and couch potato sessions, the weight gain can spiral out of control. And while everyone says it's fine because "it's just baby weight," we all know it's not the baby demanding that third helping of mac and cheese.

While pregnancy weight gain is necessary and natural, it's a delicate balance between nourishing your baby and not turning into a contestant on My 600-lb Life: Baby Edition. So, make healthy choices, keep active (as much as waddling permits), and remember: fluid retention and hormonal fat storage are temporary. The cravings, however, might stick around longer than the baby weight.

6.2. Hormones

Pregnancy weight gain isn't just about cravings or a license to eat for two; it's primarily orchestrated by hormones pulling the strings behind the scenes. Meet the stars of this biological drama: progesterone, prolactin, and human placental lactogen (HPL).

6.2.1. Progesterone

Progesterone earns its name as the ultimate pregnancy ally— literally meaning "for pregnancy." Produced by the ovaries, this hormone works overtime to ensure the fetus's survival, but not without a cost to the mother's waistline.

- **Lower BMR**: Progesterone turns your metabolism into a couch potato, conserving energy for the growing fetus. While efficient, it means fewer calories burned during even the most mundane tasks, setting the stage for weight gain.
- **Fluid Retention**: Progesterone also enjoys hoarding water like your body is a camel, leading to swelling and bloating.
- **Increased Appetite**: By stimulating hunger cues, progesterone ensures mom eats enough to sustain both

85

herself and the tiny tenant. This, combined with a lower BMR, creates the perfect storm for weight gain.

While essential, progesterone's effects make moderation in weight gain important. Excessive weight gain, thanks to its metabolic meddling, can raise risks during pregnancy and delivery.

6.2.2.   Prolactin: The Milk Mogul

Prolactin, the pituitary gland's contribution to pregnancy, is all about milk production. Its name—literally meaning "for milk"—highlights its primary goal: preparing the breasts for lactation. But there's more to prolactin than milk.

- **Fat Storage**: Prolactin encourages fat deposits, particularly in the hips and thighs, creating an energy reserve for breastfeeding. This isn't vanity padding; it's survival insurance for the baby.
- **Appetite Boost**: Like progesterone, prolactin increases appetite, ensuring enough calorie intake to support pregnancy and postpartum needs.
- **Fluid Retention**: As if water retention weren't bad enough with progesterone, prolactin joins the party, adding to bloating and weight gain.

While prolactin plays a vital role in ensuring post-pregnancy readiness, its appetite and fat storage effects make it another contributor to the battle of the scale.

6.2.3.   Human Placental Lactogen (HPL)

HPL is the hormone with a survivalist streak, ensuring that the fetus gets its due share of energy—whether or not mom is ready.

- **Sugar Liberation Expert**: HPL acts like a stress hormone, breaking down fat and releasing glucose for the fetus. This mechanism likely evolved to safeguard the baby's nourishment even during famine.

- **Gestational Diabetes Risk**: The downside? If mom overeats or gains too much weight, HPL's sugar-releasing frenzy can overwhelm the body's insulin balance. This may lead to **gestational diabetes** (GD), a precursor to T2DM later in life.

HPL's well-meaning actions, coupled with progesterone's appetite-boosting and prolactin's fat-storing tendencies, create a hormonal tug-of-war that can exacerbate weight gain.

While weight gain during pregnancy is necessary for a healthy baby and mom, hormones like progesterone, prolactin, and HPL make managing that weight a balancing act. Too much weight gain can lead to complications, including GD and long-term health risks. Working with healthcare providers and adopting a mindful approach to diet and activity can help keep hormonal hijinks in check.

6.3. Lifestyle Changes

During pregnancy, everything in a woman's life gets a makeover, from cravings that could put the cookie monster to shame to more hours spent lying down than a sloth in a hammock. And all of these lifestyle changes are here to ensure that weight gain during pregnancy doesn't just happen, but happens with style. Let's take a look at how these changes transform a woman's body, but not always in a "glow" kind of way.

6.3.1. Increased Calorie Intake

Pregnancy is a time for expansion. Not just of the belly, but also of the portion sizes. Pregnant women are often told to eat more to "nourish" the baby. And who are we to argue with that logic when it's essentially a free pass to stuff your face with food without shame? Sure, you could make healthy choices, but why do that when you can justify your third serving of mac and cheese with, *"I'm eating for two"?* Who needs moderation when you've got hormones and an excuse to eat like you're training for a competitive eating contest?

6.3.2. Reduced Physical Activity

Pregnancy also gives the perfect excuse to sit back, relax, and become a sedentary superstar. Between the fatigue, discomfort, and general feeling of being a human incubator, many women start adopting a lifestyle of *"let's just sit here and wait for the baby to do the hard work."* This means fewer calories burned, which—spoiler alert—results in weight gain. Sure, you can go for walks or do some light exercise, but why bother when the couch is so cozy and your body is busy creating a tiny human?

6.3.3. Stress and Sleep Changes

Pregnancy also introduces a cocktail of stress and sleepless nights, which somehow both contribute to weight gain. Stress, the delightful companion, triggers cortisol, which fires up your cells like a Black Friday sale. And when your brain cells are all hyped up, good luck relaxing enough to sleep. With sleep evading you like a bad ex, you're left with more awake time, which naturally means more time for eating. Insomnia: the unexpected weight-gain ally. So, while you're awake at 3 a.m. contemplating life and the size of your thighs, you're also eating your way through an entire bag of Flaming Hot Cheetos. But hey, it's for the baby, right?

6.3.4. Other Changes

Job changes, new routines, and sitting in front of the TV can also contribute to the weight-gaining extravaganza that is pregnancy. Say goodbye to the days of being active and hello to marathon Amazon Prime sessions in your third trimester. Why work when you can lounge in front of the screen, snacking and binge-watching your way through the final stretch? And let's not forget about sitting at a desk all day—it's the perfect setup for gaining weight while pretending to be productive. Who knew that career advancements and personal growth would come with a few extra pounds?

Pregnancy is all about change—and not just the baby bump. You're on a fast track to weight gain with increased calorie intake, reduced activity, stress, and sleep changes. But don't stress too much about it—this is all part of the process. Just remember to try and keep a healthy balance... or don't. After all, you've got a baby to grow, and that's an excellent excuse for an extra few donuts.

6.4. Staying Fit During Pregnancy

Exercise during pregnancy? Oh, absolutely—because growing a human isn't exhausting enough, right? Enter squats: the exercise that's equal parts functional fitness and unintentional comedy routine for the pregnant body. Let's break down why squats are your new best frenemy.

In case you've never lowered yourself to pick up a toddler or a dropped bag of snacks, squats are where you bend your knees, hips, and ankles like you're lowering yourself onto an invisible chair—except the chair doesn't exist, much like the concept of restful sleep after the second trimester.

Squats can be done with or without weights. (Spoiler: if you're pregnant, you're already carrying extra weight, so you're basically a squat champion just by existing.)

Think of squats as pre-gaming for labour. They strengthen the pelvic muscles—the unsung heroes of pregnancy that hold everything together while you slowly descend into snack-fuelled madness.

- **Pelvic Power**: Strong pelvic muscles can improve stability, reduce back pain, and, most importantly, help you avoid embarrassing waddle-related injuries. Plus, a sturdy pelvic floor might even boost your chances of a successful vaginal delivery because why not aim for a classic exit strategy for your tiny tenant?

- **Muscle Maintenance**: Squats help prevent you from tipping over like an unsteady Jenga tower as your baby grows and your centre of gravity goes rogue.

Squats don't stop being useful once the baby arrives. They help you bounce back, tone those overworked legs, and maybe—just maybe—make it easier to reclaim your pre-baby jeans. Plus, squats burn calories, which is crucial after discovering that late-night feedings are best accompanied by entire tubs of ice cream.

The American College of Obstetricians and Gynecologists (ACOG) suggests daily 20–30 minutes of moderate exercise. This can be split into shorter sessions, perfect for when you need a break from Googling "weird pregnancy symptoms" or debating the ethics of bribing your baby to sleep through the night.

As for squats, ACOG recommends doing 20–50 daily, depending on your fitness level. Start slow—because pulling a muscle while pregnant means waddling and limping.

Before embarking on your squat-filled journey, consult your healthcare provider. They'll confirm that it's safe for you and your future little gym buddy. And if anyone questions your form, remind them that you're already performing the world's most hardcore weightlifting act—growing a human life while maintaining your sanity.

Now, drop it low, mama. Well, not too low—gravity is unforgiving, and getting back up might take a while.

7. Limitations to Losing Weight

Welcome to Chapter 7, where we tackle the Herculean task of trying to lose weight—unlike Chapter 5, which was more of a *"Here's why the scale probably hates you"* pity party. Think of this chapter as the gritty reboot: same theme, darker tone, and a lot more frustration.

In Chapter 5, we explored why the universe might be conspiring against you with weight gain. Chapter 7, however, is for those poor souls making a genuine, sweat-drenched effort to shed pounds, only to discover their metabolism moonlighting as a practical joker.

Yes, there are similarities between the two chapters—you're still stuck on the same rollercoaster of dietary despair. But this chapter hones in on the specific struggles of earnest weight loss attempts, like why salads feel like you're paying reparations and why the gym smells like tears and regret.

So, buckle up and brace yourself for the brutal truth about why "serious effort" might just be the setup for a cosmic punchline.

7.1. Common Lifestyle-Related Limitations

7.1.1. Time for Physical Activity

It's the age-old excuse: *"I just don't have the time to exercise!"* Well, congratulations, you've officially joined the club of life's busiest victims. Sadly, skipping physical activity doesn't just mean you'll miss out on the thrill of sweaty boom boom and awkward gym selfies—it also means your body's calorie-burning machinery will start running on fumes.

Regular exercise boosts your Basal Metabolic Rate (BMR), helping you burn calories even when you're doing absolutely nothing—basically the closest thing to magic. Stop exercising, though, and suddenly your BMR's like, *"Okay, guess I'll nap instead."* Combine that with a sedentary lifestyle filled with binge-watching, doom-scrolling, and sitting at a desk for hours, and your metabolism waves a tiny white flag of surrender.

Stress doesn't help either. Exercise is nature's free stress reliever, but your cortisol levels skyrocket if you're too busy to sweat it out. Cortisol, the chaos-loving hormone, is like your body's overly dramatic roommate that hoards snacks in the form of belly fat.

But wait, there's more. When you're perpetually rushed, your diet becomes a tragic comedy of bad decisions: drive-thru burgers, greasy pizza, and "breakfast" consisting of a coffee and vending-machine candy bar. Spoiler alert: fast food doesn't exactly make your metabolism move faster (unless you get the left-over special from last week).

So, while you might think skipping workouts saves time, what you're really saving is calories—for your fat cells. And they'll thank you kindly by multiplying like rabbits.

7.1.2. Access to Healthy Food Options

It's the Hunger Games: Grocery Edition, where your survival depends on navigating a landscape barren of fresh produce but brimming with aisles of neon-orange cheese puffs and mystery meats. Lack of access to healthy food options is not just a minor inconvenience—it's a front-row ticket to the weight-gain carnival.

Imagine craving a crisp apple but instead finding a vending machine that offers you the choice of "Chocolate Bars" or "Potato Flakes à la Sodium." Fresh fruits, lean proteins, and whole grains? Those are mythical treasures buried deep in suburban grocery utopias, far from the food deserts where many are stranded. As a result, diets lean heavily on processed monstrosities, packed with enough unhealthy fats and added sugars to make your arteries stage a riot.

Without proper nutrients, your body becomes a sad, sluggish husk, barely burning calories while storing fat like it's prepping for a civil war. Your metabolism is basically a broken-down car at this point, sputtering, *"Feed me kale or let me die!"* And let's not forget the emotional side of this culinary tragedy.

When faced with barren shelves and greasy alternatives, frustration and hopelessness take over. Emotional eating becomes your therapist, and surprise! Your therapist is serving deep-fried everything. Stress also invites its old friend, cortisol, to the party— a hormone that gleefully stores fat like a hoarder on a reality show.

Worse still, unhealthy eating saps your energy, making simple exercise feel like an Olympic-level feat. After all, how can you hit the treadmill after a dinner of imitation cheese and sadness?

Access to healthy food shouldn't be a luxury item—it's a necessity. Tackling this issue means addressing hunger and the irony of being overfed yet undernourished. So, let's hope someone out there is lobbying for policies to replace those vending machines of doom with fresh veggie stands. In the meantime, enjoy your "carbo-loaded cry fest" with a side of existential despair.

7.1.3.   Lack of Support

Picture this: You're trying to eat a salad, and your family is waving pizza slices in your face like it's a victory flag. That's the reality when there's no squad cheering you on in your quest to lose weight—just a pitiful orchestra of emotional eating, stress, and zero motivation to lace up those running shoes.

Family and friends are supposed to be your cheerleaders, but when they're not, you might as well be running a marathon with lead weights strapped to your ankles. Without support, the stress creeps in, bringing its usual partners in crime: isolation and hopelessness. The next thing you know, you're eating a tub of ice cream because *"at least Chandler Bing never judged you."*

Oh, and let's not forget the exercise conundrum. Physical activity feels like a Herculean task when no one is there to nudge you off the couch or join you for a workout. Instead of jogging, you're binge-watching another season of Yellowstone, burning calories only with dramatic gasps during plot twists.

Lack of support doesn't just affect your morale—it actively sabotages your metabolism. No exercise means no BMR boost, no muscle gain, and no calorie burn. You're basically in a holding pattern, waiting for your body to morph into a beanbag chair.

In short, tackling weight loss without a supportive network is like fighting a dragon with a pool noodle. Sure, you can try, but the odds aren't great. So, here's hoping you find your tribe—or at least a cheesecake-free zone to focus on crushing your goals.

7.1.4. Lack of Motivation

Motivation is the mythical unicorn of weight loss—always just out of reach and prone to vanishing the moment someone mentions donuts. Without it, you're not just struggling uphill; you're crawling backward into a pit of skipped workouts and pizza boxes.

When motivation packs its bags, healthy habits become an endangered species. Suddenly, salads seem like a cruel punishment, and the treadmill? It's just a clothes rack with delusions of grandeur. You tell yourself, *"I'll start tomorrow,"* but tomorrow comes with fries, and the gym remains an untouched urban legend.

But wait, there's more. A lack of motivation doesn't just sabotage your workout schedule—it invites emotional eating to the party. Stress hits, and instead of coping like a champ, you're elbow-deep in a bag of Doritos, wondering if cheese dust counts as a vitamin. It's a vicious cycle: eat to feel better, feel worse, eat some more. Congratulations, you've unlocked the guilt buffet!

Let's be honest—without motivation, exercise is off the table, too. Couch potato status achieved. Your body? It's waving a white flag as your metabolism stalls and your muscles threaten to unionize due to lack of use.

The good news? You don't have to let the motivation void win. Set tiny goals (like not eating cake for breakfast), rope in a workout buddy, or bribe yourself with something shiny. Just remember: the journey starts with one step, preferably not into a bakery.

7.2.   Common Medical Limitations

Let's get one thing straight: this isn't about blaming your thyroid or hormones for every extra slice of cake you've eaten. Instead, this is your crash course in understanding the sneaky medical hurdles that can turn your weight-loss marathon into a slog through quicksand.

Think of these factors as the bureaucrats of your body, complicating your health goals with red tape and fine print. They're not handing you extra pounds on a silver platter (you don't get that kind of service here), but they are excellent at throwing wrenches into your progress. Hormonal imbalances, metabolic disorders, and even medications can act like uninvited party guests, making everything harder while contributing nothing positive to the vibe.

The challenge? These medical roadblocks don't show up with neon signs. They hide behind your good intentions, waiting to sabotage your calorie burn or hijack your appetite at the worst possible moments. But don't despair—this isn't about hopeless resignation. It's about knowing the enemy so you can fight smarter, not harder.

Medical factors won't pile on the pounds effortlessly, but they will make your weight-loss journey feel like an obstacle course designed by a sadist. And while I can't promise you shortcuts, understanding the lay of the land can help you navigate it without losing your sanity—or your sense of humour.

7.2.1. Certain Medical Conditions

Your endocrine system is like a drama queen of your body if ever there was one. This intricate network of hormones is like the scriptwriter for your body's metabolism, dictating how efficiently you burn calories and store fat. Unfortunately, medical conditions that mess with this system don't just cause weight gain; they also turn weight loss into the ultimate plot twist you didn't ask for.

Think of these conditions as the diva performers of your metabolism. They disrupt the harmony, hog the spotlight, and leave your healthy habits struggling for recognition. Disorders like hypothyroidism, polycystic ovarian syndrome (PCOS), or Cushing's syndrome can make losing weight feel like training for a marathon in a space suit.

Treatment? Well, it's less "wave a magic wand" and more "assemble a team of specialists and prepare for a long haul." Medication, lifestyle changes, and sometimes surgery can help tame the hormonal chaos. But here's the kicker: even with your hormones on their best behaviour, diet and exercise still take centre stage.

So, while these conditions might make your weight-management journey more like climbing Mount Everest than strolling through the park, they're not insurmountable. With the proper support and a touch of stubborn optimism, you can still rewrite the script. Just don't expect a Hollywood ending without putting in the work. See **section 5.5** for the prequel to this hormonal melodrama.

7.2.2. Medications

Some medications, like antidepressants and corticosteroids, come with the delightful bonus side effect of weight gain. It's like ordering a salad and getting fries on the side you didn't ask for. For more details on this cheery topic, check out **section 5.4.1.**

7.2.3.   Age

As the candles on your birthday cake multiply, your metabolism decides it's time to slow down, making weight loss more of a chore. Apparently, your body's idea of a gift is less muscle and more fat storage. See **section 5.6.5** for the full reality check.

7.2.4.   Genetics

Blame your ancestors—genetics can make some people naturally inclined to gain weight and fight an uphill battle to lose it. If your family tree looks more like a bakery menu, you might have inherited the weight-gain gene. See **section 5.6.1** for the DNA drama.

7.2.5.   Poor Sleep

Sleep deprivation doesn't just make you cranky; it amps up your appetite and fuels cravings for the unhealthiest foods. It's your body's way of saying, *"If you won't rest, at least feed me cookies or just the cookie dough."* Avoid this pitfall by prioritizing shut-eye. See **section 5.3.5**.

7.2.6.   Stress

Stress is a sneaky saboteur, turning your weight-loss journey into a cortisol-fuelled buffet. Emotional eating doesn't care about your calorie goals, and your body is all too eager to store those "comfort" carbs. For the gritty details, see **section 5.6.3.**

7.2.7.   Alcohol Consumption

That glass of wine or pint of beer? It's packing more calories than you'd like to admit. And if you're indulging regularly, those empty calories can quickly add up to real weight. Cheers to moderation! See **section 5.6.4** for the sobering truth.

7.2.8. Yo-yo Dieting

Yo-yo dieting is where your weight is a game of up-down-up-down, but the prize is a side of existential dread. It's like being the world's worst magician: Now you see the pounds, now you don't! Oh wait, they're back, and they brought friends.

The core problem? Consistency—or lack thereof. People lose weight, get cocky, and decide the hard work is over. Cue the weight creeping back in, like an ex who didn't get the memo. Sometimes, it's not even their fault; life just loves throwing obstacles like stress, time, and family-size pizza deals.

Fad diets promise the world and deliver…temporary misery. Sure, you'll lose weight fast—along with a chunk of your soul—but yo-yo dieting has consequences. For starters, it messes with your health in ways that would make even a fast-food drive-thru wince.

Crash diets don't discriminate—they'll burn through fat and muscle like a fire sale. And here's the kicker: losing muscle tanks your BMR. Translation? Your body becomes an expert at hoarding calories, making future weight loss feel like dragging a boulder uphill in flip-flops.

Yo-yo dieting is a hormone's worst nightmare. Cut calories too drastically, and your body responds with a cortisol spike—a stress hormone that screams, *"EAT ALL THE THINGS IN SIGHT!"* You also end up hungrier than a zombie at a salad bar, with cravings so intense you'd punch someone for a Klondike bar.

Here's the cruel twist: rapid weight loss feels like winning the lottery. But when the pounds return (as they inevitably do), motivation dies a slow, painful death. That initial high is replaced by frustration and the realization that your "health journey" is more of a post-war ordeal.

In the end, yo-yo dieting doesn't just mess with your body—it turns your relationship with weight loss into a dark comedy of errors. So, next time someone offers you the latest miracle diet, just smile and say, *"I prefer my misery without the whiplash, thanks."*

7.2.9. Inactivity

Inactivity is the secret ingredient to turning your metabolism into a slow-motion train wreck. Sitting all day like a human-shaped paperweight is not precisely the workout routine of the gods. It leads to a sluggish BMR and pitiful DEE, making your body think it's on a permanent vacation. Spoiler alert: this is not the vacation where you come back looking fit and fabulous. This is the vacation where your pants no longer fit.

7.2.10. Unhealthy Eating Habits

If you've been using a steady diet of chips, soda, and "just one more slice" of pizza as your personal nutrition plan, congratulations, you're a walking advertisement for why "fast food" should be renamed "slow death." Processed foods high in sugars, unhealthy fats, and mystery ingredients are the perfect recipe for weight gain. It's like you're trying to sabotage your own diet while giving a high-five to your future T2DM. You know you should stop, but that fourth donut is looking at you like a tragic love story. Look away and slowly back away with your tongue inside your closed mouth.

7.3. Less Common Lifestyle-Related Limitations

If you're surrounded by folks who seem to have mastered the art of these following limitations, don't panic—this doesn't mean they're taking over the planet. We're diving into the rare, almost mythical limitations people might encounter while trying to manage their weight. These are not really the unicorns of the weight loss world, but they're elusive, peculiar, and not exactly what most of us face. But hey, if you happen to be dealing with one, at least you've got a good story for your next *"What's keeping you from your goals?"* support group meeting.

7.3.1. Disordered Eating

Disordered eating isn't just about choosing a pound of kale over pizza—it's about battling mental health conditions that mess with your relationship with food and your body. We're talking about serious stuff like **anorexia** nervosa and **bulimia** nervosa, where the quest for weight loss can take a turn into dangerous territory, not just physically but mentally, too.

For anorexia, the idea is simple: fear of weight gain combined with a distorted body image leads to starvation. Sounds like a recipe for disaster, right? While it might result in weight loss (if you can even call it that when it's a life-threatening condition), it also sets the stage for a whole host of issues, like **nutrient deficiencies** and **hormonal imbalances**. And when treatment comes into play, there's a risk the pendulum might swing the other way. That once-underweight person might go full-on opposite direction, entering the world of obesity because, surprise, disordered eating doesn't just lead to underweight—it can lead to overeating too.

Then we have bulimia nervosa, where the cycle is all about binge-eating and then purging, often with self-induced vomiting or extreme exercise. While anorexia patients are underweight, bulimia patients may actually be at a healthy weight—or even overweight. But don't be fooled. Just because you're not visibly "too thin" doesn't mean the same psychological mess isn't there. When bulimia patients stop the cycle of purging and excessive exercise, what happens next? Yep, weight gain. Hormonal chaos, distorted body image, and that pesky fear of gaining weight come into play once again, making it harder than ever to stay healthy.

Let's not forget the side effects of purging: **electrolyte imbalances**, **dehydration**, and **digestive damage**—good times, right? When you engage in such extreme behaviours, your metabolism starts to freak out. It goes into "starvation mode," slowing down as it desperately tries to save energy. Once regular eating resumes, the body says, *"Hold up—let's store all this food for later, just in case!"* The result? Weight gain.

In the end, anorexia and bulimia are not just paths to temporary weight loss; they're traps that make maintaining a healthy weight a lifelong struggle. And that's on top of the health problems that come with messing with your body's natural rhythms. So, while eating disorders may look like a shortcut to losing weight, they're really just a detour to more complex issues down the road.

7.3.2.   Extreme Dieting

Extreme dieting is where the goal is to lose weight as quickly as possible, regardless of the long-term consequences. Think **drastic caloric cuts** or cutting out entire food groups—because who needs carbs or fats anyway, right? While you might drop pounds faster than a rollercoaster ride, buckle up, because this ride can end with some serious health problems.

Sure, extreme diets like juice cleanses or low-carb fads can cause rapid weight loss by slashing calories down to the bone. But here's the catch: drastic restrictions can leave your body starving for nutrients, which isn't exactly the recipe for maintaining a healthy weight.

By cutting out entire food groups, you're playing a dangerous game. No carbs? No fats? No problem, except when your body starts to cry out for essential nutrients. Missing out on vitamins, minerals, and fatty acids can leave you tired, weak, and even depressed—pretty far from the energetic, healthy person you were hoping to become.

On top of that, extreme dieting can wreck your hormones. You restrict your food, your body thinks it's starving, and suddenly, you're in a cortisol-induced panic. That stress hormone doesn't just keep you awake at night; it also tells your body to hold onto every calorie like it's a precious treasure. Add that to the mix, and you're basically begging your metabolism to go into "survival mode."

This means more hunger, more cravings, and fewer chances of sticking to a diet that feels more like torture than a lifestyle. But wait, it gets better! This vicious cycle can actually slow down your metabolism, lower your BMR, and make your DEE as low as a sloth on a lazy day. With a slower metabolism, weight gain is almost inevitable. In fact, it's the classic recipe for yo-yo dieting, where you lose weight just to gain it all back—and then some.

In short, extreme dieting might give you fast results, but it's more likely to set you up for a major fall. **Nutrient deficiencies**, **hormonal havoc**, and a **sluggish metabolism** could leave you struggling not only with weight loss, but also with your overall health. So, next time you think about cutting out food groups, maybe think twice—because extreme dieting is the fast lane to a slower metabolism and a much more challenging weight loss journey.

7.3.3.   Poor Self-Esteem

Poor self-esteem is the ultimate sabotage artist when it comes to weight loss. It's like your brain is telling you, *"Hey, you're not good enough, so let's just take it out on food!"* You start thinking that skipping meals, cutting calories, or avoiding entire food groups is the solution. Sure, you might lose weight, but not without leaving a trail of mental and physical wreckage behind.

When self-esteem takes a dive, the next stop is often an overzealous exercise routine. You think, *"If I just punish myself enough in the gym, I'll somehow earn the right to eat,"* leading to gruelling workouts that leave you drenched in sweat and possibly questioning all your life choices. Sure, you'll drop some pounds, but you'll also rack up health problems like **exhaustion**, **injuries**, and **muscle wasting** because you're treating your body like a punishment centre.

But wait—there's more! Poor self-esteem can have you ducking out of social gatherings that revolve around food. Whether it's dinner with friends, family holidays, or even birthday parties, you're avoiding these situations to dodge judgment, shame, or the simple act of eating in front of others. This only means more restriction and weight loss, but at the cost of your mental well-being and relationship with food.

However, the results of this cycle are rarely pretty. When you inevitably return to normal eating habits (because, let's face it, you can't live off celery forever), the body doesn't just say, *"Okay, cool."* It's more like, *"You deprived me for way too long; now I'm holding onto everything!"* This can lead to **electrolyte imbalances**, **hormonal chaos**, **stress-related diseases**, or—wait for it—**starvation**.

And once your body finally realizes that it's been starved for long enough, it might just reward you with a nice round of pathological weight gain, because the body loves to bounce back in the most extreme way possible. You've got yourself a real weight loss rollercoaster here, but it's not the fun kind. So, before you jump on that self-loathing express train, remember: the more you restrict and stress, the harder it'll be to maintain any weight loss in the long run.

7.3.4. Lack of Knowledge

This is a classic pitfall of not knowing what the heck you're eating. If you don't know the difference between a balanced diet and just "a bunch of stuff that's edible," you're setting yourself up for a world of weight gain confusion. Without a clue about nutrition, you might be operating under the misguided belief that cutting out entire food groups is a "surefire" way to lose weight. But news flash: you're not winning any health awards with an all-celery diet. This kind of restriction could leave you deficient in vital nutrients, low on energy, and facing the dreaded *"I can't stick to this"* feeling.

And let's talk about those processed foods you might be gravitating toward because, hey, they're "easy." Well, guess what? They're also packed with empty calories, little to no nutrients, and could soon have you wondering where your energy went, as well as adding inches to your waistline. You're essentially feeding yourself a one-way ticket to weight gain, high blood pressure, and

103

possibly an invitation to the heart disease party.

But it gets even juicier. Without proper nutrition knowledge, your idea of portion control might resemble that of a bottomless pit. *"Oh, this bowl of pasta is just one serving... or, you know, maybe three."* If you have no clue how much you should be eating, chances are you'll be eating more than your body actually needs, quietly sabotaging your weight loss goals with each unsuspecting bite.

So, it's high time to educate yourself if you're still guessing the difference between good and bad fat (hint: it's not about whether it's deep-fried). A little knowledge goes a long way toward making healthier food choices, keeping portion sizes in check, and, just maybe, finally breaking free from the weight gain cycle. Your body—and your waistline—will thank you later.

7.4. Less Common Medical Limitations

7.4.1. Hormonal Imbalances

Hormonal imbalances, like an overactive thyroid or insulin resistance, can totally mess with your weight loss journey. Your hormones are supposed to be working together like a well-choreographed dance, but when one of them decides to go rogue, things can get ugly. Whether it's an overactive thyroid that speeds up your metabolism (but makes you feel like you're running on fumes) or insulin resistance that leads to pesky weight gain around your belly, these imbalances can create serious roadblocks in your quest for a slimmer you. It's time to get those hormones in check if you want to see some real progress. See **section 5.4.2** for more.

7.4.2. Malabsorption

Malabsorption is when your body becomes a terrible host and refuses to absorb nutrients properly. It's like your small intestine has a VIP section, but only certain nutrients are allowed in, and it's a strict "no carbs" zone. Whether it's because of celiac disease,

Crohn's disease, cystic fibrosis, or even a surprise guest like worms in your stomach (yay, party!), this condition can lead to weight gain in some delightfully ironic ways:

- **Increased Calorie Intake**: Since your body is basically throwing out the VIP pass for nutrients, you end up needing to eat more food just to get the basics. More food = more calories = more weight. It's like your stomach is a bottomless pit, but not in a fun, buffet sort of way.
- **Reduced Energy Expenditure**: When your body can't get the nutrients it needs, it's like trying to run a car on empty—no fuel, no function. Your body decides, *"Why bother with exercise? Let's just store all these leftover calories as fat and call it a day."* BMR and DEE take a nap, and your waistline gets the memo.
- **Increased Insulin Resistance**: Because your body can't handle insulin properly (thanks, malabsorption), it gets all grumpy and spikes your blood sugar. The result? Your body's like, *"Well, I guess I'll just store all these excess calories as fat then. Thanks, malabsorption!"*
- **Hormonal Imbalances**: Malabsorption's gift to you? A cortisol boost. And what does cortisol do? It makes you hungry. Because if there's one thing you need when you're not absorbing nutrients, it's definitely more food. Great.
- **Water Retention**: Because why not throw in some water retention for fun? Malabsorption can cause your body to hoard fluid like it's preparing for a drought. So, suddenly, you're heavier and squishier, and that's not even including the weight from your soul-crushing existential crisis.

In short, malabsorption is like your body's version of a bad roommate—it takes what it wants, ignores your needs, and leaves you picking up the calories (and water weight) it didn't want. Enjoy the ride!

7.4.3. Chronic Pain

Chronic pain is like that annoying guest who never leaves the party and slowly takes over your life. This persistent pain lingers, affecting everything from your mood to your ability to walk without looking like a penguin on crutches. And guess what? It's also great at contributing to weight gain. Here's how:

- **Less Physical Activity**: Chronic pain can turn even the simplest tasks, like walking to the fridge, into an Olympic sport. And let's be honest: if you're spending more time hugging the couch than lifting weights, your muscle mass and metabolism take a nosedive. The result? Your body starts storing extra fat as if it's preparing for some kind of survivalist retreat.
- **Impact on Daily Activities**: Things you used to take for granted, like cooking dinner or grocery shopping, suddenly feel like a Herculean feat. When you're too exhausted or in pain to get off the couch, it means less physical activity, which means more calories hanging around uninvited.
- **Food and Stress**: Let's not forget about the emotional rollercoaster. Chronic pain often brings along stress and anxiety, which is fantastic for making you crave comfort food. And when stress and chips go hand in hand, you can bet that your diet goes out the window. The result? You're eating all the wrong foods and packing on those extra pounds, because who can resist a chocolate bar when you're miserable and in pain?

In short, chronic pain is like a weight-gaining conspiracy. It slows you down, messes with your food choices, and leaves you with more weight than you signed up for. At least it's consistent, right?

8. Fundamental Principles

Achieving and maintaining a healthy weight is a noble quest—like slaying the dragon of temptation while dodging the flaming arrows of excuses. The following principles can be your trusty sword and shield, assuming you're not battling any debilitating medical or lifestyle limitations. Used together and consistently, these strategies might work (yes, even if you're convinced your metabolism is powered by disappointment and regret). Embrace them, and you just might see visible, long-term results—provided you don't get sidetracked by a well-timed cheesecake.

8.1. Reduce Your Total Calorie Intake

The eternal battle of "calories in versus calories out" boils down to a simple truth: what you eat versus what your body burns determines whether your waistband stays loyal or stages a rebellion. If you eat more than your body needs, you'll gain weight. If you eat less, you'll shed pounds—assuming you can outlast the siren song of pizza and cookies.

Each pound of fat is worth a hefty **3,500 calories**. That's right; your body hoards energy like a doomsday prepper. To lose a pound, you need to create a 3,500-calorie deficit. Conversely, scarf down an extra 3,500 calories, and congratulations, you've gained a pound—probably while binge-watching a series about healthy living.

Your daily caloric needs depend on age, gender, weight, activity level, and whether you believe dessert is mandatory. For instance, your basal metabolic rate (BMR)—the calories you burn just staying alive—is **24 times your weight in kilograms**. Translation: even lying down, you're a calorie-burning machine (just a very, very slow one).

Say you're 220 lbs (100 kg). Your BMR is 24 x 100 = 2,400 calories/day. Add in how much you move (or don't) to get your Daily Energy Expenditure (DEE). If you're a couch potato, multiply by 1.3. If you're running marathons for fun (who hurt you?), multiply by 1.7. If you're somewhere in between, multiply by 1.5.

For instance:

- DEE for a 220 lbs (100 kg) couch potato: 24 x 100 x 1.3 = 3,120 calories/day (because couch-flipping channels is effort).
- DEE for a 165 lbs (75 kg) Marathon Enthusiast: 24 x 75 x 1.7 = 3,060 calories/day (now that's commitment).

If you consume exactly your DEE, you'll maintain your current weight. Exceed it, and you'll gain weight. Stay below, and you'll lose it—unless your metabolism files for early retirement. Many medical and lifestyle factors can affect your DEE.

To lose weight, you can either eat less or move more. Ideally, both—because why choose one form of suffering when you can have two? Let's say you're munching 3,500 calories/day, and your DEE is 3,000 calories/day. Cutting 500 calories a day means you'll likely lose 1 pound in a week.

Alternatively, you could slash 10% off your intake for a gentler approach. Cutting 350 calories daily means losing 1 pound every 10 days. Just skip your morning muffin—or, you know, that entire sleeve of Oreos.

Aim for a weight loss of less than 1% of your body weight per week. Anything more veers into crash-dieting territory, and trust me, you don't want to set up camp there. Also, your metabolism (a.k.a. the moody teenager of bodily functions) might not always cooperate, thanks to age, gender, or some ancient grudge it holds against you.

8.2. Reduce Eating Empty Calories

Empty calories are the junk mail of the food world. They're flashy, tempting, and utterly useless. Sure, they provide energy, but when it comes to nutrients like fibre, vitamins, and minerals, they're about as helpful as a chocolate teapot. Think sodas, sugary snacks, and cakes—they pack a caloric punch but leave your body crying for real sustenance.

Most empty-calorie foods are sugar bombs. Sugar, a simple carbohydrate, rockets into your bloodstream, spiking your blood sugar like a rollercoaster without the fun. Insulin jumps in to shuttle sugar into cells, storing it as liver glycogen, muscle glycogen, or—surprise, surprise—fat. The cycle continues since fat storage has unlimited capacity (thanks to evolution).

Here's the kicker: a can of pop (200 calories) leaves your stomach faster than an excuse to skip the gym, making you hungry for more. But a bowl of cereal with the same calories? That can keep you full for hours. Hypothetically, you could guzzle 10 cans of pop (2,000 calories) in a few hours and still have room for dessert. Sound familiar?

Frequent sugar binges don't just overwork your pancreas; they send insulin levels into overdrive. Over time, your pancreas might throw in the towel, leaving you with sky-high blood sugar and a VIP pass to complications like Insulin-dependent DM, heart disease, strokes, or worse. Sudden death? Now, that's a dramatic plot twist we'd rather avoid.

Empty-calorie foods also tend to be loaded with unhealthy fats—trans and saturated varieties—that clog arteries and increase the risk of heart disease. These fats are like the shady characters of your diet, quietly wreaking havoc while sugar takes all the blame.

Instead of letting empty calories rob you blind, focus on whole, unprocessed foods. Trade that soda for water or herbal tea. Swap the cake for a piece of fruit. And hey, if you must indulge, practice portion control. Remember, sharing that slice of cake saves calories and might make you a friend for life.

Snacking? Sure, but make it count. Reach for a handful of nuts or a satisfying veggie instead of a candy bar. And remember, moderation isn't just a buzzword—it's your best defence against an empty-calorie takeover.

In the end, it's okay to indulge occasionally. Just don't let empty calories take up permanent residence in your diet. Your body deserves better, and deep down, you know it.

8.3. Increase Your Fibre Intake

Let's talk about fibre, the indigestible saint of your plate. It's a carbohydrate found in fruits, veggies, legumes, and whole grains that strolls through your stomach like a tourist, refusing to be digested. While other carbs bend over backward to give you energy, fibre is too busy minding its business and improving your health in the most passive-aggressive way possible.

Fibre has a unique talent: it slows your stomach's emptying time. Translation? You stay full longer. It's like a bouncer at a nightclub, keeping your appetite in check so you don't dive headfirst into a snack drawer at 10 p.m. Studies even show that eating more fibre can lead to modest weight loss. So, think of fibre as that friend who subtly reminds you to put the cookie down without the judgmental side-eye.

Fibre doesn't just hang out; it takes on cholesterol with the kind of dedication that should win awards. When dietary fat teams up with bile salts to help your intestines do their job, fibre says, *"Not so fast, buddy."* It binds to those bile salts, dragging them out of your body like an embarrassing party guest. Your body, ever the overachiever, is forced to make more bile salts. Since bile salts are made from cholesterol and cholesterol can be made from body fat, more fibre in your diet means burning through cholesterol and even stored fat. Eat more fibre, and you'll have cholesterol running for the hills faster than a middle-aged man at the sight of commitment.

Fibre comes in two flavours—soluble and insoluble—and both have their quirks. **Soluble fibre**, the water-loving gel-former, is the overachiever. Found in oats, beans, and fruits, it lowers cholesterol, regulates blood sugar, and keeps you feeling full. **Insoluble fibre**, the rough-and-tumble sibling, doesn't dissolve in water. Instead, it bulks up your stool, ensuring your bathroom visits don't turn into existential crises. Whole grains, nuts, and fruit skins are its stomping grounds.

Together, they're like a mismatched buddy-cop movie—soluble fibre plays the smooth-talking negotiator, while insoluble fibre handles the dirty work.

The recommended daily fibre intake is 25 grams for women and 38 grams for men, but let's be honest—most of us are falling short. To fix that, you can:

1. Toss some fruit and veggies into your meals.
2. Choose whole grains like a responsible adult.
3. Invite beans and lentils to your culinary party.
4. Snack on nuts and seeds (or at least pretend to enjoy them).

But fair warning: don't go from zero to fibre hero overnight unless you want your stomach to stage a protest. Gradually increase your intake and hydrate like you're training for a marathon.

In the end, fibre isn't here to be your best friend—it's here to keep you alive and slightly less of a hot mess. So, give it the respect it deserves. After all, fibre doesn't just improve your health—it might also save you from eating an entire bag of chips in one sitting. Maybe.

8.3.1. Eat Cereal Every Morning

Cereal is probably humanity's greatest invention after fire and sarcasm (I'm still not impressed by sliced bread). One glorious benefit of starting your day with a bowl of cereal is that it helps you feel full or at least tricks you into thinking you're full. The secret weapon? Insoluble fibre. This miraculous substance is nature's version of packing peanuts—it doesn't break down and bulks up your stool like a champion. Congratulations, your colon just became a bodybuilder.

Feeling full is crucial, especially if you're trying to manage your weight (or avoid eating the entire contents of your fridge by 10 a.m.). Let's say you eat cereal at 8 a.m.; by some lovely twist of biology, it might hold you over until 10 a.m. That's two whole hours of not thinking about donuts. Progress!

Cereal can also bully cholesterol into submission if feeling full wasn't enough. Many cereals come fortified with plant sterols, which are like tiny cholesterol ninjas. They sneak into your bloodstream and block cholesterol absorption. Your body doesn't even see it coming.

The real MVP in this story? Bile salts. These little guys help digest fats and generally mind their business—until fibre shows up and binds to them, forcing them to hitch a ride out of your body via your colon. To replace the exiled bile salts, your body raids its cholesterol reserves. Goodbye, cholesterol! Hello, smug sense of dietary superiority.

Cereal rarely flies solo; it has milk, the Robin to its Batman. Not only does milk hydrate your sad, shrivelled soul, but it also brings calcium to the party. Calcium builds strong bones, helps your heart beat, and gives your nervous system something to brag about. Plus, it helps synthesize bile salts, so you can keep that cholesterol-lowering cycle going.

Not all cereals are created equal. Some are so loaded with sugar they might as well be dessert. Pro tip: if your cereal comes with a cartoon mascot, maybe you should pay attention to the sugar content. Opt for something high in fibre and low in sugar—because there's no pride in getting outsmarted by the same cereal that impresses a 4-year-old.

Sure, milk has sugar and cholesterol, but fibre in cereal more than makes up for it. Fibre doesn't just regulate bowel movements and lower cholesterol—it's also your digestive system's way of telling you, *"I got this."* So, pour yourself a bowl of cereal, sit back, and enjoy knowing your breakfast is doing the heavy lifting—literally. Just don't forget to thank your colon later.

8.3.2.   Eat an Apple After Every Meal

Eating an apple after every meal might be the easiest health hack since someone decided that running when no one was chasing you was a thing. With around 4 grams of fibre per apple, you're knocking out a good chunk of your daily fibre goal (15% for women and 10% for men) every time you chomp down one. It's like your digestive system gets a round of applause for every bite.

Fibre doesn't just make your bowels happy; it's your secret weapon against cholesterol. Think of it as a bouncer that grabs the extra cholesterol hanging around your bloodstream and kicks it out. Left unchecked, cholesterol can build up in your arteries like rush-hour traffic, leading to heart attacks and strokes. No one wants their arteries to feel like a congested freeway.

Need more fibre intel? Review the intro to this section. Spoiler alert: your gut will thank you.

But wait, there's more! Apples are packing **vitamin C**, the **antioxidant** that fights free radicals—those rogue molecules that damage cells and try to ruin your day (and your health). Vitamin C swoops in like a superhero, neutralizing free radicals and leaving your body feeling invincible.

Vitamin C also helps produce collagen, which keeps your skin looking youthful and your gums healthy. No one wants to revisit the 18th century and scurvy, where collagen breakdown led to tooth loss, and pirates learned that eating citrus was not evil.

And let's not forget your immune system. Vitamin C **boosts white blood cell production**, making sure your body is ready to slap down germs faster than you can say, *"Pass me another apple."*

Apples also bring a sweet hit of fructose, nature's way of saying, *"Here's an energy boost, but don't go crazy."* Unlike candy bars, apples won't leave you crashing faster than a cheap website, or a cheap drunk at a bachelorette party.

Adding an apple to your post-meal ritual might seem like a minor move, but it's a stealthy health revolution. You're not just eating a fruit—you're helping your body manage cholesterol, regulate blood sugar, ward off disease, and stay collagen-rich.

So, next time you finish your meal, grab an apple. Your arteries, immune system, and future self will thank you. And who knows? Maybe you'll even start saying, *"An apple after every meal makes you look so hot that the doctor can't keep away (wink, wink)."* Okay, maybe not, but it's worth a shot.

8.3.3. Increase Your Vegetable Consumption

Veggies are the unsung heroes of your plate. A vegetable-rich diet isn't just a health trend; it's the MVP of good living. These leafy, crunchy, colourful wonders bring a buffet of benefits that your body can't help but cheer for. Let's dig into why veggies deserve all the hype.

Vegetables are like the bouncers of the cholesterol world. Thanks to cellulose, they help escort bile salts out of your body like an unwanted guest, leading to lower cholesterol levels. Fewer bile salts mean less cholesterol hanging around, which means a reduced risk of heart disease. Think of veggies as your heart's personal security detail.

Vegetables can give it a much-needed wake-up call if your metabolism feels like it's on a never-ending vacation. Power-packed greens like broccoli and spinach are loaded with nutrients that can crank up your BMR. Translation? You burn more calories just by existing. Who knew sitting on the couch could be so productive?

Vegetables are basically nature's multivitamins. With heavy hitters like vitamins A, C, and E, they wage war against free radicals, those pesky molecules that age you faster than a bad relationship. Want youthful skin, a strong immune system, and super-powered cells? Start piling on the greens.

Before you cook your veggies to oblivion, remember that not all nutrients enjoy the heat. Vitamin C is a drama queen—it's water-soluble and heat-sensitive, meaning it can vanish faster than your willpower in front of a chocolate cake. Overcooking also destroys folate (vitamin B9), leaving you with a side dish of sadness instead of a nutrient powerhouse.

Pro tip: Lightly steam or sauté your veggies to keep the vitamins alive and kicking. Your body—and your taste buds—will thank you.

Eating more vegetables is like hitting the jackpot of health. Veggies do everything from lowering cholesterol to boosting your metabolism and arming you with essential nutrients. Just don't overcook them, or you'll turn your health jackpot into a soggy consolation prize.

So, make it a point to toss more greens into your meals. Your waistline, heart, and future self will give you a standing ovation.

8.3.4. Include at Least Two Salad Snacks Every Day

Salads are the superheroes of healthy eating—easy to assemble, brimming with nutrition, and a sneaky way to eat your vegetables without feeling like you're munching on a garden. Eating raw veggies in a salad isn't just convenient; it's like giving your body a VIP pass to all the vitamins and nutrients cooking might otherwise destroy.

Packed with vitamins, minerals, and antioxidants, raw vegetables can help you dodge chronic illnesses like heart disease, T2DM, and certain cancers. And let's not forget fibre—the unsung hero that keeps your digestion on track and prevents those awkward *"I-haven't-gone-in-days"* moments.

And the calorie count? Minimal. Fat content? Practically non-existent—unless you accidentally drown your greens in creamy ranch. (Don't worry, I'll get to dressing soon.)

When building your salad, go full Monet: the more vibrant, the better. Red tomatoes, orange carrots, and green spinach don't just look pretty; they're antioxidant powerhouses. Think of each colour as a different health benefit, like collecting bonus points for your body.

Now, let's talk salad dressing—the potential villain of this otherwise virtuous meal. Opt for unsaturated oils, like olive oil, which is basically liquid gold for your heart. Rich in monounsaturated fats, olive oil can lower cholesterol, improve blood sugar control, and even give T2DM a run for its money.

But remember, olive oil prefers to stay raw. Cook it, and it loses some of its charm. Drizzle it straight onto your greens and enjoy the guilt-free flavour upgrade.

Adding two salads a day to your routine is like giving your body a health makeover. It's low effort, high reward, and a surefire way to up your veggie intake without turning on the stove. Just don't overdo the dressing, or you might turn your salad into a dessert in disguise.

So, grab a bowl, toss some veggies, and give yourself a crunchy pat on the back.

8.4. Replace Calorie-dense Foods with Healthier Choices

We've all heard it: Breakfast is the most important meal of the day! (Followed by Lunch is a good idea; Dinner can ruin your figure; and Midnight snacks are a cry for help.) But seriously, breakfast is like the first step in your daily survival strategy, giving you the nutrients and energy to avoid turning into a cranky, hangry mess by noon. And if you're looking to manage your weight without feeling like you're fasting for Lent, skip the calorie bombs and opt for a nutrient-dense breakfast instead.

Let's start with plantain—a banana that's basically trying to be a potato and failing miserably, but we love it anyway. It's a starchy carbohydrate that releases energy slowly. That's right, no sugar rush followed by a shame spiral at 10 a.m. Plantains give you a steady flow of energy, like a drip-feed for your body that keeps you from face-planting into your desk. They're also packed with potassium, which is excellent for your heart and muscles. Because we all know you need something to keep you standing after two hours of pretending to work.

Next up: eggs. These little protein bombs are like the Swiss Army knife of nutrition. They've got everything: muscle-building amino acids, healthy fats, and enough cholesterol to make your arteries do a happy dance (just kidding—don't push your luck). But seriously, eggs are great because they give you that "full" feeling, meaning you won't be diving into your colleague's lunch leftovers by 10:30 a.m. Not to mention, when paired with plantains, the protein and fat balance out those slow-release carbs. It's like a symphony in your stomach.

Let's talk about tomatoes, the fruit masquerading as a vegetable. They're loaded with vitamin A (for your skin, teeth, and eyesight—basically all the things you ignore until they fall apart) and **lycopene**, a powerful antioxidant that makes tomatoes look so red and sassy. Lycopene's job is to beat up free radicals in your body into submission. So yeah, a little tomato slice is basically giving cancer the middle finger.

Avocados, the overpriced green mush, somehow became the symbol of "self-care." They're full of healthy fats—monounsaturated fats, to be exact—they love to lower your cholesterol. Plus, they've got vitamin E, which keeps your skin looking like you are in love for the first time, and gives your immune system the strength to fight off whatever cold your coworker brought in. And don't forget the fibre—so you can keep your digestive system running like a well-oiled machine. You know, until your next cake binge.

And what's the best way to wash down all this goodness? Water. The magical elixir that keeps you alive. Sure, you can opt for fresh juice, but don't kid yourself, it's just sugar water with a vague vitamin C label on it. Either way, hydration is key, especially when you're about to power through your inbox without collapsing into a caffeine-fuelled coma.

Now, let's compare. You could go for the classic breakfast of four slices of bread (380 calories), two fried eggs (392 calories), and a cup of coffee (because obviously). That's about 800 calories, and guess what? It's basically bread and fried fat. Good luck with the vitamins—there are none.

Or, you could go for a breakfast that's actually worth your time: One plantain (122 calories), two boiled eggs (310 calories), avocado (160 calories), tomato (11 calories), and a glass of orange juice (120 calories). Total calories: 720. You're saving 80 calories, but more importantly, you're getting fibre, nutrients, and minerals that will keep you full for twice as long without the post-bread crash.

So, here's the moral of the story: Opt for the plantain, eggs, avocado, and tomato combo—your body will thank you. The bread breakfast? It'll probably make you want to nap under your desk by noon. And let's be honest, you've got enough of that going on already.

8.5. Reduce Red Meat Consumption

Red meat—beef, lamb, pork, or whatever other animal you're cooking—has been a staple protein source for as long as we've had fire. But before you go diving into that juicy steak, here's a little reminder: too much of it can be a health nightmare in disguise. So, let's talk about why moderation is key when it comes to your red meat intake.

Despite being a protein powerhouse, red meat is also a fat powerhouse—and we're talking saturated fat here, the kind that raises your cholesterol levels like a bad reality TV show can raise your blood pressure. The more you chow down on fatty cuts of red meat, the more likely you are to increase your total cholesterol, making your heart and arteries regret your life choices. Too much of this stuff can lead to heart disease and strokes. So, to avoid those heart attacks, cut back on the steak and take your arteries out for a nice, low-fat date.

Now, onto iron. Red meat is packed with it, and while iron is crucial for transporting oxygen through your blood and keeping your immune system in check, there's such a thing as too much of a good thing. If you're munching down on steak every night, you could be putting yourself at risk for iron overload, a condition that makes your body store more iron than it knows what to do with. This can lead to liver damage and a higher risk of certain cancers—so, you know, not ideal. Men, especially, are more prone to this since they don't have the monthly "iron purge" that women do. So, unless you want your body to turn into an iron storage facility, maybe consider scaling back the meat.

Reducing red meat can be an easy win if you're trying to shed a few pounds or maintain a healthy weight. Red meat is calorie-dense, so reducing your intake will automatically lower your overall calorie consumption without having to count every bite of food like you're on a diet reality show. If weight loss or maintenance is your goal, trimming the red meat might be just what the doctor wants—unless your doctor is secretly a butcher, in which case, run.

Okay, now that you know why you should lay off the red meat, let's talk about how to do it without feeling like you've been sentenced to a life of bland salads. You don't have to go full vegan

119

(unless you want to), but here are some ideas:

- **Beans and Lentils**: They're like the protein superheroes of the plant world—cheap, tasty, and full of fibre.
- **Seafood**: It's got protein, omega-3s, and all the good stuff you need without the guilt.
- **Lean Cuts of Red Meat**: If you're not ready to break up with red meat, at least go lean and trim off any excess fat.
- **Processed Meats**: Bacon, deli meats, and sausages are fun in the moment, but they're the sodium-loaded, preservative-filled villains of the meat world. **Limit them**.

Red meat isn't the enemy—it just shouldn't be your diet's headliner. Consumed in moderation, it has its place in your diet, especially for those who need a little extra iron. But if you want to keep your cholesterol in check, your iron levels from turning into a metal factory, and your weight from going off the rails, it's time to add some variety to your protein game. Red meat has benefits, but mixing it up with plant-based proteins, seafood, and leaner cuts is better. After all, there's a world of flavours beyond your favourite fatty steak. You just have to be willing to explore it.

8.6. Space your Dinner Time from Bedtime

So, you're hungry at midnight and debating whether that leftover pizza or that tub of ice cream will be your late-night salvation. Spoiler alert: That snack could sabotage your health—and your waistline. If you're scarfing down dinner less than four hours before hitting the hay, you're setting yourself up for some serious fat storage, not the kind you want.

When you eat late, especially right before bedtime, your body doesn't exactly put those calories to good use. You're about to enter the world of sleep—where you turn into a human-sized sloth. Your body goes into "idle" mode, making those calories less likely to be used for energy. Instead, they get stored away as fat in your cozy little fat cells. This delightful process is called lipogenesis—when your body turns excess glucose into fat because it has no energy demands to satisfy. Nice, right?

Now, glucose is your body's primary source of fuel, but if you're not moving around, that fuel just sits there, building up. So, if you're munching on carbs late at night, they'll turn into fat faster than you can say, *"Oops, I ate a second slice of cake."*

We all know that feeling—one bite turns into five, and suddenly, you've eaten an entire extra-large pizza without realizing it. But here's the kicker: It's way easier for your body to turn those carbs into fat than it is to burn through the fat it already has, hence the saying, *"A moment on the lips; forever on the hips."* Your metabolism slows down while you're sleeping, and those calories you consumed late at night are just begging to be stored for later use. Sorry, but your body isn't exactly in fat-burning mode when you're snuggled in bed, dreaming of all the snacks you could be eating.

And don't even get me started on digestion. Eating a huge meal right before bed is like asking for a digestive disaster. Your body produces stomach acid and enzymes to break down food, but when you're lying down, gravity isn't doing its job. Those digestive juices have nowhere to go but up your esophagus, which can result in heartburn, indigestion, and that oh-so-comfortable feeling of misery. So much for sweet dreams.

But wait—don't worry, you don't have to suffer through a night of hunger pangs. If you're craving something before bed, opt for fresh fruit. Not all carbs are created equal, and the fructose in fruit is efficiently digested by your body, even when you're just lying there like a potato. This means the calories from fruit are less likely to be stored as fat—your body actually has a way of using them even in sleep mode. Plus, they won't disrupt your digestive system and send you into the bellyache zone.

If you're serious about avoiding the dreaded weight gain, it's time to swap your late-night snacks. That bowl of ice cream and a slice of cake? Yeah, no. Instead, grab an apple, a handful of strawberries, or some other fresh fruit. Your body will thank you, and you'll wake up feeling a lot less like you swallowed a boulder. Eating better and smarter before bed? Now, that's a snack strategy worth keeping.

8.7. Stay Hydrated

Let's talk about hydration, the unsung hero of literally every bodily function. Forget your fancy diets or hardcore gym sessions—if you're not guzzling water like a fish with an existential crisis, you're sabotaging yourself. Dehydration doesn't just leave you thirsty; it slowly transforms your body into a malfunctioning mess of fatigue, cramps, and mental fog so dense that you'll forget why you walked into a room for the fifth time today. Still, you have no idea why you walked into that room. No, it's not Alzheimer's; you're probably just dehydrated.

When you're dehydrated, your body gets a little... confused. Instead of burning fat for energy, it decides, *"Hey, let's eat muscle instead!"* Great plan, right? Because nothing screams "healthy weight management" like cannibalizing your own gains. Proper hydration keeps your metabolism on track, so your body torches fat instead of the muscle you worked so hard to build. Skip the water, and your weight loss journey becomes a tragic Shakespearean drama—except no one claps at the end.

Think of electrolytes as your body's Wi-Fi connection—when it's strong, everything works. When it's weak? Welcome to Buffering Central. Dehydration messes with this delicate balance, leaving you with cramps that make you look like you're auditioning for a zombie flick. Proper hydration, however, keeps those electrolytes happy and your organs functioning. It's not glamorous, but neither is collapsing into a puddle of regret and Gatorade.

Burning calories is like hosting a wild party in your body: it's fun while it lasts, but someone's gotta take out the trash. That "trash" is waste products from calorie burning, and without enough water to flush it out, you're left with a toxic mess. Hydration is your body's janitor—silent, underappreciated, but absolutely necessary. Skip it, and your insides start resembling a hoarder's garage.

But good news! Fruits are here to save the day, hydrating you while tasting like happiness. Fruits are packed with water, electrolytes, and vitamins like multi-tools for your health. Bonus: They also have fibre, so you can go number two like a champion. Forget the overpriced electrolyte drinks—just grab a watermelon and start gnawing.

If regular water isn't doing it for you, there are fancy options like coconut water or electrolyte drinks. Sure, they're pricier than tap water, but your body is a luxury car, right? Might as well give it premium fuel. Just don't replace actual meals with these drinks unless you're going for the "starving marathon runner" look.

Basically, hydrate or die. Okay, maybe not die, but you'll undoubtedly suffer in ways that make dehydration feel like a villain in a bad horror movie. Drink water, eat fruit, and keep your body functioning like the semi-competent adult you're pretending to be. Because the alternative? A tragic cycle of fatigue, bad decisions, and muscle loss. Don't be that person. Drink the damn water.

8.8. Learn to Savour Your Food

Ever get that greedy, *"I need to stuff my face"* feeling? We've all been there. The challenge is that your food doesn't magically teleport to your stomach the moment you swallow it. It's not just gravity doing the job; your food pipe, or esophagus if we're getting fancy, has smooth muscles that do a little dance every time you swallow. If those muscles don't groove properly, swallowing becomes tricky. When you munch away, your conscious control takes a back seat the moment you swallow, and the unconscious part of your nervous system grabs the wheel.

As your stomach fills up, it stretches. When it hits max capacity, your stomach shoots a message to your brain saying, *"Hey, we're full, buddy, stop eating!"* If your brain doesn't get the memo or decides to play the rebellious teenager, you might end up on a caloric rollercoaster. Ignoring your stomach's *"I'm full"* message and continuing to eat is what we call **cortical overdrive** – your cerebral cortex, the brain's control centre, takes over, ignoring your stomach's pleas for a ceasefire.

Now, imagine your brain getting the *"I'm full"* text late. Picture this: you're famished, contemplating devouring a whole cow. You sit down, start inhaling food, and here's the catch – only the food in your stomach can send the "I'm good" message to your brain.

By the time that satisfaction signal reaches your brain, your stomach has hit its maximum stretch. However, your food pipe (esophagus) is still delivering food. This surplus food may further push your stomach's stretch limit, creating a new "maximum." And guess what? Over time, you'll need more food to reach that "full" sensation. Keep this up, and you're on the express train to Weight Gain City.

To avoid this slippery slope, you must be mindful of what you eat and how you eat it. Speed eaters take note: savour and enjoy your food. Slowing down means less food in your stomach and esophagus and less stretching overall. Taking your sweet time while eating makes it unlikely that any food will linger in your esophagus when your stomach shouts, *"That's it, I'm full!"*

This technique isn't just about being a foodie; it's a stealthy way to reduce your calorie intake. Taking your time chewing your food (some recommend masticating (not the other word) at least 10 times before swallowing) and waiting a mere 10 seconds after you swallow anything before another bite can work wonders.

Want to level up? Wait 10 seconds before sipping water or a low-calorie beverage, then 10 more seconds before taking another bite. That water might add to the total volume entering your stomach, nudging it to max capacity earlier. Thanks to the volume added by water or another low-calorie beverage, your stomach may max out with fewer calories.

So, instead of battling calories head-on, become a food connoisseur. Enjoy each bite, take your time, and inadvertently, your calorie intake will play a quieter tune. It's not just about eating less; it's about savouring more!

8.9.   Stop or Reduce Alcohol Intake

Alcohol, the elixir of bad decisions and extra belt notches. Let's break it down, shall we? Drinking in moderation might not sabotage your swimsuit season, but go overboard, and you're not just drinking spirits; you're summoning the Ghost of Waistlines Future.

Every shot, beer, or wine glass you lovingly cradle might as well whisper, *"I'm 150 calories closer to your stretchy pants!"* Alcohol is the king of empty calories, meaning it gives you energy but not a single nutrient. It's like a Tinder date that only talks about CrossFit: initially entertaining, but ultimately useless.

Your liver, the overworked and underappreciated detox factory, treats alcohol like an annoying coworker who demands attention immediately. While it's busy metabolizing that vodka soda you just had to have, it neglects other responsibilities, like burning fat. The result? Fat gets stored—probably in places you least want it. Thanks, tequila.

Drinking boosts insulin production, which basically tells your body, *"Hey, let's hoard some fat!"* Combine that with alcohol-induced cravings for fries or an entire pizza, and you're basically planning a coup against your own metabolism.

Ever notice how a couple of drinks turns you into a bottomless pit of hunger? That's ghrelin, your hunger hormone, throwing a wild party in your stomach. That's why your "just one drink" night ends with you spooning Nutella straight from the jar while contemplating your life choices.

As if the calorie parade wasn't bad enough, alcohol also messes with how your body handles carbs. Instead of using them for energy, your body starts stashing them away as fat—like a squirrel hoarding nuts for the apocalypse.

Alcohol doesn't just lower your inhibitions; it lowers your standards for a date, food and movement. Drinking turns *"I'll just have a salad"* into *"Bring me all the nachos in Mexico,"* and your gym session into a long nap interrupted only by brunch plans.

Moderation is key—because blacking out and packing on pounds is a terrible combo. Stick to lower-calorie drinks, balance your buzz with water, and maybe don't let margaritas peer-pressure you into inhaling three baskets of poutine. Your liver—and your jeans—will thank you. See **section 5.6.4.** for more.

8.10. Maximize Workouts with Effective Timing

Exercise is like a good relationship: timing is everything. Work out at the wrong time, and your body will punish you with cramps, sluggish digestion, or, worse, an existential crisis about why you even got out of bed. Let's unpack the science behind this sweaty saga.

Your body's primary goal during digestion is to prevent you from dying from undigested pizza. When you exercise too soon after eating, your muscles hijack the blood meant for your stomach, leaving you with cramps and a regret-fuelled treadmill session. The solution? Wait at least two hours after your meal before exercising, unless you enjoy playing *"Will I Vomit, or Won't I?"*

Your hormones are like moody gym coaches. Cortisol, the stress hormone, peaks in the morning, yelling at your fat cells to burn, baby, burn. Testosterone, the multitasking hormone, also shows up early, ready to boost muscle gains and improve performance. Morning workouts, then, are the overachiever's choice—burning stored calories after that 10-hour overnight fast. Plus, avoiding your boss's "urgent" 8 a.m. email is a solid excuse.

Here's the good news: no matter the time of day, exercise reduces your chances of heart disease, T2DM, and looking like a human potato. But there's a catch. If you have uncontrolled hypertension or your chest decides it's auditioning for a medical drama, you might want to consult a healthcare provider. When it's painful for your body, please don't force it. No means no.

Exercising before bed is like texting your ex at midnight—it can feel good but might mess with your sleep. Sure, it's great for muscle gains and stress relief, but don't blame the treadmill when you're lying in bed at 2 a.m., wide awake and questioning your life choices.

Exercise timing matters, but it's not the be-all, end-all. Pair your perfectly timed workouts with a balanced diet, quality sleep, and the occasional rest day (Take a cheat day with a Netflix marathon). After all, a healthy lifestyle is about balance—between your muscles and your stomach, your hormones and your schedule, and, most importantly, between you and that tempting slice of cheesecake.

8.11. Divide Your Exercises into Muscle-building and Cardio-intensive

So, you've decided to tackle weight management, and now you're facing the eternal fitness question: Should I lift heavy things repeatedly or run nowhere for 30 minutes? Let's break it down so you can make an informed (and slightly less sweaty) decision.

Building muscle isn't just about looking good in tank tops. When you pump iron or conquer resistance bands, you're turning your body into a calorie-burning machine. Here's why:

- **BMR Boost**: Muscles are calorie-hungry. More muscle means a higher BMR, which is like having a furnace that

127

burns calories while you're binge-watching a documentary about body positivity.

- **Efficient Energy Storage**: Muscles store glucose as glycogen, keeping it handy for energy instead of sending it off to fat storage. Think of it as your body's *"friends don't let friends store fat"* program.
- **Improved Insulin Sensitivity**: Resistance training keeps your insulin working harder than a new in-law at a family reunion, reducing blood sugar and fat storage while improving your body's fat-burning efficiency.

Bonus: You may also gain the ability to carry all your groceries in one trip.

Cardio, the OG of fat-burning, is like the unsung hero of exercise. It doesn't get as much credit for building muscles, but boy, does it get your heart pumping and your fat crying. Here's what cardio brings to the table:

- **Fat Targeting**: Cardio forces your body to dig into its fat reserves like it's rummaging through a junk drawer for batteries. It's particularly good at eliminating the "stubborn fat" that loves to cling to thighs and bellies like an overzealous toddler.
- **Heart Health**: Want to avoid becoming a walking heart attack waiting to happen? Cardio's got you covered, reducing your risk of heart disease and T2DM while giving your heart the workout it deserves.
- **Mental Perks**: While a runner's high might not be as cool as Wi-Fi, it's a close second for improving mood and reducing stress.

Hydration is key whether you're lifting, running, or awkwardly pretending to stretch while scrolling Instagram. Dehydration can sabotage your workout and leave you feeling like a shrivelled raisin. Drink water—lots of it—no excuses.

The best weight management strategy isn't choosing sides but playing to both strengths. Want to burn calories while you rest? Build muscle. Want to torch stubborn fat while pretending you

128

enjoy jogging? Do cardio. The real magic happens when you combine the two.

Now, go forth and conquer the gym, the living room floor, or wherever your workout adventure begins. Just remember to hydrate—and maybe treat yourself to a celebratory smoothie afterward. You earned it.

8.12.   Work on Your Cardio Before Weight Training

Starting an exercise routine can feel like trying to pick a Netflix show—too many options, and none of them sound fun. Do you dive into cardio or head straight for weight training and risk looking like a baby giraffe trying to deadlift? Spoiler alert: start with cardio. It's like the entry-level fitness job—necessary, humbling, and pays in sweat instead of money.

Let's face it: your heart's been coasting for years. Cardio is like telling your heart, *"Hey buddy, it's time to earn your keep."* Whether you're jogging, cycling, or flailing in a pool like a confused otter, cardio makes your heart work harder. Over time, it gets stronger and learns not to panic when you chase after a bus or attempt stairs.

Think of cardio as a training montage for your lungs. As you huff and puff, your body becomes a pro at using oxygen efficiently. This is crucial for weight training, where your muscles demand oxygen like toddlers demand snacks. Without it, you'll be wheezing in a corner while the gym bros stare. With it, you'll be lifting longer, harder, and possibly even with fewer existential regrets.

Cardio is the calorie-burning superhero your muffin top never asked for. A good run or bike ride doesn't just torch calories—it cranks up your BMR (Basic Metabolic Revenge) so your body keeps burning calories even when you're binge-watching shows later. And when you start weight training? Those extra calories go straight to repairing your muscles, not sticking around like unwanted party guests.

Let's be real: starting an exercise routine can be as stressful as meeting your partner's parents for the first time. Cardio helps by turning your stress into sweat. Whether it's pounding pavement or cycling to nowhere on a stationary bike, you'll leave feeling lighter (mentally) and slightly deader (physically). Plus, it's a great way to build the confidence you'll need when you inevitably drop a dumbbell on your foot later.

Cardio is the gateway drug to fitness. It prepares your heart, lungs, and fragile self-esteem for the chaos of weight training. Gradually, you'll work your way up from "barely surviving a brisk walk" to "owning the weight room like a mildly awkward champ." So, lace up your shoes, put on your playlist, and remember: no one looks fabulous on their first treadmill run. But they all look cooler than the guy who didn't try.

8.13. Do Less Intensive Workouts but More Frequently

The "more is better" mantra doesn't always apply when building muscle. Sure, you could spend four hours in the gym trying to Hulk-out in one day, but your body will reward you with crippling soreness, muscle tears, and a deep sense of regret. Turns out, doing less (and more frequently) is not just smarter—it's also a great excuse to avoid the gym bros who live there.

Picture your muscles as overworked interns. Every time you exercise, you're essentially saying, *"Hey, do more!"*—and they comply, tearing themselves apart in the process. But if you don't let them rest, you'll have mutiny, leaving you weaker and more broken than a New Year's resolution. Skip the overkill, and give your muscles the time they need to repair. Like fine wine, gains take time—unless you're okay looking like a soggy noodle forever. Long, intense workouts build lactic acid, the gym's version of revenge. It leaves you sore, tired, and questioning every life decision that brought you here. Keep your workouts short and sweet; lactic acid won't have time to move in and ruin your life. Less lactic acid = fewer mornings where you can't climb stairs without looking like a newborn giraffe.

You can't just pick up the heaviest dumbbell and expect to become a superhero overnight. That's how you get crushed. Instead, slowly increase your weights or reps over time. This lets your muscles adapt without filing a complaint to HR (or your physical therapist). Think of it as upgrading your torture device gradually—it's less horrifying that way.

The real secret to gains? Science says to chill. Overtraining doesn't make you tougher; it makes you tired, sore, and prone to injuries. Frequent, less intense workouts are like YouTube binges for your body—manageable, consistent, and oddly effective.

So, the next time you're tempted to annihilate your body in one marathon session, remember: your muscles hate you, but they hate stupidity more. Doing less-intensive workouts more frequently will build muscle, avoid injury, and keep your soul intact. Or as intact as it can be when squats are involved.

8.14. Reduce Heavy Workouts

Classic gym flex: slapping 200 lbs. on the bench press and feeling like a Greek god for 45 seconds. While that's great for your fast-twitch muscle fibres (and your ego), it might not do much for your calorie-burning ambitions. If weight loss is the goal, it's time to delve into the fascinating world of muscle fibres, where science meets sweat.

Fast-twitch fibres are the gym equivalent of high-maintenance party guests—they show up, make a dramatic impact, and leave before the real work begins. These powerhouses excel at short bursts of intensity, like lifting heavy weights or sprinting. But their energy strategy is... inefficient. They guzzle glycogen like frat boys at a keg party, leaving your fat stores virtually untouched during your workout.

So, while you're crushing that 200-lb. bench press, your fast-twitch fibres are essentially saying, *"Great party, but we're out of snacks!"*

Enter slow-twitch fibres, the laid-back endurance champs. They're like your friend who jogs for fun and still has the energy to go hiking afterward. These fibres are smaller, slower, and much better at burning fat because they use oxygen more efficiently. Lighter weights and higher reps wake these fibres up, allowing them to flex their calorie-burning superpowers.

Translation: Want to burn fat and boost your metabolism? Maybe ditch the 200 lbs. for a set of dumbbells that don't double as a small child.

Here's the twist: your BMR is doing most of the calorie-burning work anyway, even when you're sprawled on the couch, questioning your life choices. By targeting slow-twitch fibres, you can increase your BMR, effectively turning your body into a slightly more efficient calorie-burning machine. It's like upgrading from a flip phone to a smartphone—you'll notice the difference.

Look, I'm not saying you should abandon heavy lifting altogether. Fast-twitch fibres still have their perks, like building strength and making you look like a superhero in tank tops. But mixing in higher reps with lighter weights keeps your slow-twitch fibres happy and your metabolism buzzing.

All this talk about muscle fibres won't matter if you still eat an entire pizza after your "light workout." Calories in versus calories out is the harsh, unfunny punchline of fitness. So yes, eat the pizza, but maybe save the crust for tomorrow.

Your body is a muscle fibre democracy, and both fast- and slow-twitch fibres have their roles. Alternate between heavy lifts and lighter, high-rep workouts for a balanced approach that builds strength and burns fat. Oh, and don't forget the diet—your slow-twitch fibres can only do so much if you're outpacing them at the buffet.

8.15. The Power of Squats

Squats are the leg-burning, sweat-inducing exercises that make you question your life choices whenever you lower yourself onto a chair the day after leg day. Beyond sculpting buns of steel and thighs that could crush watermelons, squats might be your secret weapon in managing high blood sugar. Yes, those gruelling reps are pulling double duty.

Here's the deal: your glutes, the MVPs of your lower body, are glucose-guzzling machines. Unlike most tissues that rely on insulin to take up sugar, your glutes are rogue agents—they can grab glucose straight from your bloodstream, no insulin required. Think of them as sugar bounty hunters: the bigger and stronger they are, the more glucose they can burn.

So, if you're dealing with high blood sugar, squats can turn your posterior into a sugar-destroying powerhouse. Bonus? You'll also look fantastic in jeans.

Squats do more than just give your legs a workout. Targeting the glutes, quadriceps, and hamstrings engages large muscle groups that demand more energy. This creates a "sugar sink" effect, where glucose is pulled from your bloodstream into these hardworking muscles. It's like turning your body into a metabolic black hole for carbs.

If the idea of blood sugar control isn't thrilling enough, consider this: squats are your best defence against aging like a rusty tin man. Thigh strength is the unsung hero of staying upright as you age, reducing the risk of falls and preserving mobility. Want to be the cool grandparent who dances at weddings? Do your squats.

Now for the elephant in the room (or, rather, the junk in the trunk). Squats will give you stronger glutes but may also give you bigger ones. If that's not your aesthetic, don't panic—balance your squat routine with other exercises. Just remember, bigger glutes mean better sugar-burning.

While squats are great, they're not a magical cure for high blood sugar. You'll still need a balanced approach: eating right, taking prescribed medications, and monitoring your levels. Squats are like the cherry on top of your healthy lifestyle sundae.

Squats are the Swiss Army knife of exercises: they build strength, improve mobility, and help manage high blood sugar. Plus, they make your glutes the envy of your gym buddies. But don't just take my word for it—consult your healthcare provider before diving headfirst into squat city. Your future self, with killer thighs and well-regulated blood sugar, will thank you.

8.16.   Never Lose > 1% of Your Weight per Week

Weight loss is the eternal struggle between wanting to look like a Greek god and realizing you'd sell your soul for a cheeseburger. Let's pause if you're in the *"Let's lose it all in a week"* camp. Because if you sprint to Skinny Town, your body might just file for divorce.

Lose weight too fast, and your body's hunger hormones go feral. Leptin, the *"I'm full, please stop eating"* hormone, takes an extended vacation. Enter ghrelin, your body's devil-on-the-shoulder whispering, *"Eat the cake. Eat all the cake."* The result? A ravenous monster ready to devour an entire buffet while crying over Fitbit stats.

Lose weight slowly, though, and you trick your body into thinking it's just making lifestyle upgrades rather than prepping for an apocalypse.

Drop pounds too fast, and your gallbladder might stage a rebellion in the form of gallstones—tiny, stone-like shards of pure agony. They form when your body can't keep bile (in your gallbladder) in liquid form, thanks to a cholesterol-to-bile salt ratio that's more unbalanced than your ex's text messages.

The process is simple:

1. Lose weight fast, and cholesterol levels drop too quickly.
2. Bile salts, the lazy overachievers of the body, don't ramp up production.
3. Your gallbladder mutters, *"Screw it,"* and starts throwing stones.

If you're a fibre fanatic, you might think, *"Fiber helps me lose weight and stay regular—what's not to love?"* But surprise! Fibre also eliminates bile salts, the very thing preventing your gallbladder from becoming a rock tumbler. Translation: even your kale smoothie might be out to get you.

Quick weight loss doesn't just mess with your body—it also wrecks your mental state. One minute, you're strutting in skinny jeans; the next, you're sobbing into a pint of ice cream because the weight came back like a bad sequel.

The psychological toll? Crippling self-doubt, plummeting motivation, and the realization that you'll need therapy and a bigger belt. Slow, steady weight loss avoids this emotional whiplash, leaving you smugly sipping green tea while others cry into their cheat-day fries.

Losing weight at a snail's pace might not get you Instagram-ready overnight, but it'll save you from a raging gallbladder, hunger-induced meltdowns, and emotional collapse. Besides, life's too short to spend it battling gallstones or falling victim to yo-yo dieting.

So, embrace the slow burn. Your body (and your bathroom scale) will thank you. You could also try avoiding kale smoothies for a while.

8.17. Slowly Build Your Momentum

Making significant changes to your life can feel like trying to teach a cat to do your taxes—overwhelming, confusing, and likely to end in tears. But fear not, because the secret to success isn't about rushing into the deep end without a floatie. It's about slowly building momentum so you don't crash and burn before you even start.

Trying to do everything at once? That's the fastest way to get a one-way ticket to Injury Town or Burnout Boulevard. If you go from couch potato to marathoner in a single bound, expect your body to file a lawsuit for emotional distress. Likewise, if you slash your calories like you're on a mission to be a walking skeleton, don't be surprised if you end up crying into a packet of chips 24 hours later.

Gradual progress allows your body to adjust without needing a full-blown intervention. Start small, build up, and let your body play catch-up. That way, when your muscles start to ache, you can say, *"I earned that!"* instead of sobbing, *"Why do I hate myself?"*

If you try to drastically cut out entire food groups, your body will panic like a cat in water. Not only will you feel sluggish and hangry, but you'll also be dangerously close to pulling a *"What's the point?"* moment. Instead, focus on small, manageable changes. Start swapping processed snacks for healthier options; it's not like you're prepping for a three-day juice cleanse. You're building a lifestyle, not an emergency.

When you ease into things, you'll give your body time to adapt and strengthen itself, so you're not chasing results in a way that leaves you feeling disappointed or cranky.

Let's be real: Making life changes too fast is like a bad relationship. One minute, you're on cloud nine; the next, you're crying over spilled milk and wondering where it all went wrong. Overloading yourself with expectations will have you ready to throw in the towel before you've even gotten to the good part. But if you pace yourself and focus on bite-sized goals, you'll gradually build confidence and motivation, turning those *"I can't"* moments into

FOR PROPER AND EFFECTIVE WEIGHT MANAGEMENT

"Look what I just did!"

As you reach these small wins, your mental state will thank you. Feeling less like a failure and more like a superhero is way more fun, don't you think?

At the end of the day, changing your lifestyle isn't just about looking fabulous for your next selfie. It's about making lasting habits that will keep you feeling good long after the initial excitement wears off. Sure, it takes time to develop a balanced routine, but every bit of effort pays off when your new habits become second nature. Not to mention, you might actually add a few extra years to your life—so you can finally beat your parents at something.

No one said change was easy, but implementing a dozen life-altering habits in a day is a recipe for failure. Instead, incorporate a few minor changes at a time—your future self will thank you when you're not crying over your new, overly restrictive diet. And while each of these strategies might help independently, the real magic happens when you combine them. So, whether you're seeking help or figuring it out yourself, remember: slow and steady wins this marathon, my friend.

9. Tips for a Balanced Life

So, you've decided to embark on the extraordinary odyssey of weight management. Bravo. Welcome to the land of kale smoothies, overpriced gym memberships, and a deep, unrelenting hatred for people who say, *"Have you tried intermittent fasting?"* This isn't just about shedding pounds; it's about trying not to lose your mind while society tells you how to "fix" yourself.

Weight management isn't a "one-and-done" deal. Nope. It's a lifelong shift, kind of like that time you bought a houseplant and realized you'd signed up for years of guilt-ridden watering schedules. This isn't a quick fix; it's a permanent existential crisis with a side of salad.

But don't worry. It's not just about the numbers on the scale; it's about figuring out how to eat a cookie without spiralling into shame while secretly plotting the downfall of the person who brought donuts to work.

If you think you're about to survive on lettuce and air, think again. This is about balance. You can still have a cupcake, but first, you must eat quinoa so dry it feels like chewing on sandpaper. Moderation is key—or so they say while you side-eye your fridge at 3 a.m., wondering if cheese counts as a vegetable.

Exercise isn't just about getting fit; it's about discovering new and exciting ways to hate yourself. First, you'll try jogging while questioning every decision you've ever made. Then, you'll hit the gym, where strangers grunt loudly while you stare at the machines like alien artifacts.

But hey, after a few weeks, you might start liking it. Or you'll just be too numb to care. Either way, progress!

Let's not pretend this journey is all rainbows and protein shakes. You'll have bad days when all you want is to crawl into a blanket fort and eat an entire cheesecake. And that's okay. Your mental health is just as important as your physical health—probably more, considering how much brainpower it takes to figure out if almond milk is worth the hype. So, be kind to yourself—or at least less mean.

At the end of the day, weight management is about more than looking good in skinny jeans. It's about feeling good, having energy, and living long enough to outlast your enemies. This isn't a sprint; it's a marathon.

Celebrate the small victories, laugh at the ridiculous moments, and don't take it all too seriously. After all, life is too short to count every calorie—but just long enough to regret that third slice of cake.

Now, go forth and conquer your journey, one awkward burpee and questionable smoothie at a time. Good luck—you're going to need it!

9.1.   Keep A Food Diary For At Least One Month

When it comes to managing weight, step one is brutally honest self-awareness—a bit like reading your old Facebook posts, except this time it's about what you eat. To truly understand your eating habits, you'll need to track every meal, snack, and sneaky midnight fridge raid. Welcome to your food diary, where judgment is optional, but enlightenment is guaranteed.

Start by listing everything you eat and drink—yes, even that handful of chips you stole from a co-worker. Jot down meal times, portion sizes, and every condiment (looking at you, ranch dressing). You'll notice patterns, like skipping breakfast or inhaling cookies at 3 p.m. like it's a competitive sport.

Tracking your meals is like uncovering a food-based whodunit. The culprit behind those extra pounds? Hidden calories. That "healthy" smoothie? Basically a milkshake in a yoga outfit. And don't even get me started on coffee creamers; they're sugar bombs masquerading as harmless additions.

Go old-school with a notebook, or embrace the tech gods with apps that scan barcodes and calculate macros. Some apps even cheer you on for eating a carrot—because, hey, validation is everything. But remember, this isn't about calorie obsession. It's about catching the culprits behind your snack drawer's depletion.

Stick with this for a month, and you'll see patterns emerge. Maybe you're a serial breakfast skipper or an overzealous condiment enthusiast. Whatever the case, this diary will reveal the truth. Use this knowledge to adjust your habits, like eating a balanced breakfast or realizing that mayo doesn't belong on everything.

A food diary isn't about shame; it's about power. Knowing what you consume empowers you to make mindful choices. It's like therapy for your diet—with fewer tears and more fibre. So, embrace your food diary. It's your ticket to better health, fewer regrets, and maybe even discovering you don't actually hate kale.

Start your food diary as soon as you start hating your love handles. Who knows? It might just turn you into the mindful eater you always pretended to be.

9.2. Identify the Junk or Unnecessary Foods in Your Diet

Taking a good, hard look at your diet can be like inspecting a stranger's cart at the grocery store: enlightening, cringeworthy, and full of questions. But fear not—this step is essential for healthier eating habits. First, let's face the villain of your culinary tale: junk food.

These calorie-packed saboteurs may infiltrate your diet:

- **Soda and sugary coffee drinks**: Liquid desserts in disguise.

- **Chips, cookies, and candy**: Delicious, sure, but they're basically empty promises wrapped in salt and sugar.
- **Processed snacks**: Easy to grab, easier to regret.

Let's be real. Junk food is convenient, tasty, and always there for you—unlike your ex. But it's also sabotaging your health and weight goals. The solution? Ghost it. Replace that daily soda with water or unsweetened tea. Swap out chips for nuts or fruit, and make peace with whole-grain crackers instead of cookies. It's a glow-up for your pantry.

Rome wasn't built in a day, and your junk food habits won't vanish overnight. Start small. Replace one snack at a time, and don't look back. Soon, you'll find yourself snacking on almonds instead of chips and wondering how you ever thought neon-orange cheese dust was a food group.

This isn't a temporary breakup; it's a divorce, a lifestyle change. You'll pave the way for long-term success by ditching junk and embracing healthier options. And who knows? Maybe you'll even stop craving that bag of chips after dinner (or at least crave it less).

So, here's to a future filled with mindful eating, fewer sugar crashes, and maybe a little less shame when you peek into your snack stash. You've got this!

9.3. Set a Goal to Reduce/Eliminate These Foods from Your Diet

Congratulations! You've identified the junk in your diet. Now, it's time to do the impossible: set goals to reduce or eliminate it. Think of this as staging a dietary intervention—for yourself.

Let's get specific. Vague goals like "eat healthier" won't cut it. Instead, aim for something like:

- "No junk food on weekdays." (Weekends can be cheat

days; no one's judging.)

- "Limit junk to 10% of my diet." (Because math makes everything better.)
- "Replace one unhealthy snack per week with a healthier option." (Baby steps, folks.)

Specific goals = accountability. And accountability = fewer late-night chip binges. Don't set goals that make you miserable. If you vow to give up all junk food forever, you'll either fail or cry over your kale salad while your friends eat fries. Start small:

- Ditch sugary drinks this month.
- Swap one snack for a handful of almonds (they're fancy and nutritious).

Progress over perfection is the mantra.

Survived Monday-Friday without soda? You're basically a superhero. Picked an apple over that vending machine candy? Nobel Peace Prize-worthy. Celebrate your victories—whether with a happy dance, a gold star, or smugly telling your friends how healthy you're becoming.

Dietary perfection is a myth. Slip-ups happen. Maybe you devoured a donut after swearing off sugar—so what? The key is to keep going. Small, consistent changes lead to significant, sustainable results.

So set those goals, track your progress, and don't forget to laugh along the way (preferably with your mouth full of celery sticks instead of cookies). This journey isn't about deprivation; it's about becoming the best version of yourself—one realistic goal at a time.

9.4. Improve Access to Healthier Alternatives

So, you've ghosted junk food (mostly). Now what? It's time to meet your healthier rebound snacks—the nutrient-packed options that don't just taste good but also care about your well-being.

Apples, bananas, and berries are like the wholesome best friends you never knew you needed. They're sweet, full of fibre, and won't call you at 3 a.m. to wreck your diet. **Pro Tip**: Pair apple slices with peanut butter. It's basically a hug for your taste buds.

Almonds, cashews, and pistachios are rich in healthy fats and protein, making them the snack equivalent of that overachieving kid in high school. **Warning**: Stick to small portions. Nuts are calorie-dense, so don't turn a "healthy handful" into a "Netflix-fuelled avalanche."

Not only is yogurt high in protein and calcium, but its probiotics are like little gut cheerleaders, rooting for your digestive health. **Pro Tip**: Choose plain yogurt and add your own fruit or honey. Flavoured versions often have more sugar than a candy bar.

Carrot sticks, cucumber slices, and bell pepper strips dipped in hummus are like the cool, healthy couple at a party—they're perfect together and make everyone else look bad. Rice cakes or whole-grain crackers are a blank canvas for delicious toppings. Smear on some avocado, nut butter, or a dollop of hummus, and you're basically a snack artist.

Snack Survival Tips:

- **Plan Ahead**: Keep a stash of nuts, fruits, or crackers in your bag.
- **Out of Sight, Out of Mouth**: Don't leave chips and candy lying around. Make junk food work hard to find you.
- **Batch Prep**: Chop veggies or portion nuts ahead of time. You're less likely to binge on junk when the healthy stuff is grab-and-go.

If you find yourself face-first in a bag of chips, don't panic. It's a snack, not a scandal. Acknowledge it, forgive yourself, and grab a handful of almonds next time.

Over time, you'll notice junk food loses its appeal. Why? Because these healthier alternatives are tasty, satisfying, and—unlike that bag of cookies—they won't ghost you when it's time to fit into your jeans.

9.5.   Plan Ahead

Let's be real—if junk food had a motto, it'd be, *"I'm always here when you're not prepared."* But guess what? With a bit of planning, you can turn the tables on those greasy temptations.

Think of a weekly meal plan as your junk food kryptonite. Take 30 minutes each weekend to map out your breakfasts, lunches, dinners, and snacks. Bonus points if you make a grocery list so you're not wandering the snack aisle like a lost soul.

Never leave the house without backup. A piece of fruit, a handful of nuts, or veggies with hummus in your bag can be the difference between devouring a granola bar and raiding the nearest vending machine.

Meal prep isn't just for gym bros and food influencers. Chop those veggies, portion those nuts, and batch-cook your meals. Future You will thank Present You when dinner takes five minutes instead of 50.

Planning protects your waistline and saves your wallet. With a shopping list in hand, you'll avoid buying the "family-size" chips that were never meant for one person.

Let's face it—life happens. And sometimes, that slice of pizza or chocolate bar will win. The trick is to let it be a rare indulgence, not a ritual for every day that ends with y.

When you've got healthy meals and snacks ready to roll, junk food loses its edge. Plus, sticking to your goals will make you feel like the responsible adult you swore you'd never become.

So go ahead, plan like a boss, and show that bag of chips who's in charge. **Spoiler**: It's you.

9.6. Review Your Food Diary at the End of Each Week

Congratulations, you've survived another week of documenting every bite, sip, and late-night snack you swore was "just one." Now comes the fun part: playing detective with your food diary.

First, comb through your food diary like it's a crime scene. Do Fridays scream "pizza and regret"? Do you snack like a raccoon when stressed? These patterns aren't just quirks—they're clues.

If weekends are when your diet takes a vacation, prep your defence. Stock up on healthier options or plan meals in advance. You'll thank yourself when Sunday rolls around, and your "dinner" isn't three slices of leftover cheesecake.

If you notice you've been inhaling chips every time your boss emails you, it's time for a new coping strategy. Try meditation, exercise, or screaming into the void—whatever works.

Writing down "entire bag of gummy worms" in your food diary hits differently than mentally pretending it never happened. Seeing it in black and white keeps you honest and, let's face it, mildly horrified.

This isn't about self-loathing or guilt-tripping yourself over that second slice of pie. It's about being honest with yourself and using that data to build a more thoughtful plan for the future.

Use these insights to adjust your diet, manage your triggers, and keep moving toward your goals. Think of your food diary as your cheat sheet for life—minus the actual cheating.

Remember, you're not aiming for perfection—just progress. And next week, when the gummy worms call your name, you'll know better. Probably.

9.7. Seek Support from Your Loved Ones

Making lifestyle changes for weight loss is like embarking on a quest—except instead of magical swords, you've got kale smoothies and gym shoes. And every hero needs a squad to cheer them on (or at least stop waving cookies in their face).

Your first move? Recruit your support team. Tell your family and friends about your goals, and how they can help. Translation: *"Please, for the love of all things holy, stop ordering pizza every Friday night!"* Having your loved ones on board can make a massive difference, even if they just swap the chips for carrot sticks every now and then.

Pro tip: Rope them into your journey. Convince your friends to join your workouts—because sweating together builds bonds, or something like that. And if you can't persuade them to do burpees, at least get them to help with meal prep. Nothing says love like someone chopping veggies for your bland but healthy stir fry.

Celebrate the small wins, too. Lost a pound? Managed a workout without dying? Share your progress with your squad—they'll be your cheerleaders (minus the pom-poms). And when setbacks happen (because they will happen), they'll remind you that it's not about perfection—it's about progress.

So, rally your troops, set your sights on victory, and remember: the right support system can make even the toughest weight-loss journey almost bearable.

FOR PROPER AND EFFECTIVE WEIGHT MANAGEMENT

9.8.   Do Not Rely on Quick Fixes

Losing weight is like trying to solve a Rubik's cube while blindfo-

lded—challenging but not impossible. The trick? Forget the quick-fix shortcuts that promise miracles but deliver disappointment. Instead, think marathon, not sprint. Small, sustainable changes are your golden ticket to long-term success.

Start simple: add more fruits and veggies to your plate, bid farewell to processed foods and sugary drinks (they're just drama in disguise), and move your body in ways that make you feel like the main character in a workout montage. Over time, you can level up your exercise game as your stamina improves—baby steps, not boot camp.

Pro tip: Stop comparing your journey to someone else's highlight reel, especially the Instagram kind where lighting and filters work harder than the gym itself. Focus on your goals, your progress, and your vibe.

And hey, don't be a lone wolf. Seek support from a healthcare pro or personal trainer who understands that your path is unique. Together, you can craft a plan that's as personalized as your Spotify playlist.

Patience, persistence, and a sprinkle of self-love? That's your recipe for success. Now, go rock that journey like the champion you are.

9.9.   Get Enough Sleep

Sleep is the unsung hero of weight management—your secret weapon for staying on track. When you skimp on sleep, your body turns into a hormonal rollercoaster, cranking up ghrelin (the hunger hormone) and dialling down leptin (the appetite suppressant). The result? You're left craving that extra slice of pizza when you'd usually say no.

But wait, there's more! Sleep deprivation doesn't just mess with your appetite—it also zaps your energy and motivation, making it harder to crush your workout or even lace up your sneakers. On the flip side, getting enough sleep keeps you energized, clear-headed, and ready to make healthier choices throughout your day.

Aim for 7–9 continuous hours of quality sleep each night to supercharge your weight management journey. Need tips? Try these:

- Stick to a consistent bedtime routine, even on weekends.
- Skip the late-night lattes and wine (if you need wine to sleep, you might have another problem).
- Create a cozy, distraction-free sleep zone (yes, that means putting your phone to bed too).

Remember, rest is just as important as eating kale or doing squats. So, treat your sleep like the VIP it is—your body (and waistline) will thank you!

9.10.   Eat More Vegetables

Adding more vegetables to your diet doesn't mean turning into a rabbit—it's about upgrading your meals with flavour, variety, and nutrients.

Visualize this: at least 50% of your plate as a veggie haven. Add a side salad, a mix of roasted broccoli and carrots, or even a heap of sautéed spinach to your meals. Breakfast fan? Toss spinach into your omelette or avocado slices onto your toast.

Make your meals a feast for the eyes and body by picking vibrant vegetables. Carrots and red peppers for beta-carotene, leafy greens for iron and calcium, and purple cabbage for antioxidants. A colourful plate means a broader range of nutrients.

Thankfully, boiling isn't your only option. Roast veggies with olive oil, grill them for a smoky flavour, or sauté them with garlic and herbs for a quick, delicious side dish. A dash of balsamic glaze or a sprinkle of Parmesan cheese can turn simple veggies into a gourmet treat.

This isn't about banishing carbs or protein; it's about balance. Vegetables should complement your other food groups to create meals that are as satisfying as they are healthy.

From weight management to disease prevention, eating more vegetables fuels your body with fibre, vitamins, and antioxidants. Plus, their low-calorie nature means you can fill up without filling out.

Challenge: At your next meal, make it colourful and veggie-packed. Your plate—and your body—will thank you.

9.11.   Limit Your Intake of Sugary Drinks

What you drink is just as crucial as what you eat to maintain a healthy lifestyle. Sugary beverages like soda, sweetened coffee drinks, and sports drinks are calorie-packed and nutrient-poor, contributing to weight gain and other health risks.

These beverages are a sneaky source of empty calories and added sugars that offer no real nutritional benefits. Excess consumption can lead to weight gain, blood sugar spikes, and an increased risk of chronic conditions like T2DM and heart disease.

Better Beverage Choices:

- **Water**: The ultimate go-to. It's calorie-free, hydrating, and essential for every bodily function.
- **Infused Water**: Add lemon, mint, cucumber, or berries for a splash of natural flavour.

- **Unsweetened Tea**: Rich in antioxidants, tea can be enjoyed hot or cold for a refreshing alternative.
- **Freshly Squeezed Juice**: A vitamin-packed option, but consume in moderation due to natural sugars.

How to Transition:

- **Swap Gradually**: Replace one sugary drink per week with water or tea.
- **Read Labels**: Look for "100% juice" with no added sugars when buying bottled juice.
- **Pre-Plan**: Carry a water bottle to stay hydrated and resist the urge to grab a sugary alternative.

The Benefits?

- Reduced calorie intake
- Improved hydration
- Stable energy levels
- Long-term health improvements

Challenge: For the next week, make water your primary beverage. You'll notice a difference in your energy and overall well-being. It's a small change with big rewards!

9.12.　Choose Healthier Snacks

Snacking is one of life's greatest pleasures, second only to complaining about people who take up two parking spots. But when choosing snacks, it's less about what you want and more about what won't leave you questioning your life choices at 3 a.m.

Let's start with the good stuff. Fresh fruits like apples, bananas, and berries are great snacks because they're sweet, full of fibre, and don't judge you for eating them in bed. Plus, they come in nature's original packaging—no unholy plastic wrappers reminding you that the planet is doomed.

Nuts are like that one friend who's super supportive but also a little too expensive to hang out with. Almonds, walnuts, and cashews are loaded with protein, fibre, and healthy fats. But here's the catch: eat too many, and suddenly, you've consumed enough calories to fuel a small army. Also, if you grab the salted ones, enjoy your bloated, sodium-soaked reflection in the mirror.

Whole grain crackers and rice cakes are the Switzerland of snacks: neutral, safe, and mildly satisfying. They crunch, don't bite back, and keep your calorie count from spiralling into the abyss. Just make sure they're the real deal—whole grains, minimal sugar, and none of that "mystery ingredient" nonsense that sounds like a villain in a sci-fi movie.

Now, let's talk about the bad guys. Chips, cookies, and candy bars are the toxic exes of the snack world—irresistible, but they'll ruin you. High in sugar, fats, and guilt, they're the snack equivalent of asking your dentist if caramel counts as a vegetable. Sure, they taste amazing, but so does the thrill of bad decisions, and we know how those turn out.

The next time hunger strikes, don't let your inner gremlin talk you into inhaling a bag of chips. Instead, reach for something that won't send you spiralling into existential dread about your arteries. Choose wisely, snack thoughtfully, and remember: every healthy choice is one less regret to mull over during your next sleepless night.

9.13. Make Gradual Changes

Changing your diet can feel like climbing Mount Everest—without Sherpas, gear, or even a clue as to why you're doing it. But good news! You don't need to sprint to the summit. In fact, it's better to shuffle your way there like a reluctant teenager heading to a family reunion.

If dessert is your love language, don't ghost it—ease out of the relationship. Eating two servings a week? Cut it to one. Once you've survived that heartbreak, reduce further, maybe to once every other week. You're not giving up; you're "creating space to grow," like every toxic relationship advice column says.

Love processed snacks? Of course you do. They're crunchy, salty, and engineered to override your better judgment. But you can stage a rebellion. Replace one junk snack a week with something healthier, like fruits, nuts, or whole grain crackers. Soon, you'll barely miss those chips—until you walk past the snack aisle and hear them calling your name. Stay strong.

The secret to a diet that works? Trick yourself into not realizing you're on one. Too many changes at once can make you crack faster than a cheap smartphone screen. Stick to minor tweaks, like swapping soda for water or sneaking veggies into your meals like a stealthy culinary ninja.

Healthy eating isn't about crossing a finish line but not collapsing on the track. Celebrate small victories, like not eating that second cupcake or choosing carrots over cookies (even if it hurts a little). Progress is progress, even if it's slow.

Start small, stay sneaky, and remember: this is a long game. Celebrate every step forward because every healthy choice brings you closer to a you who can smugly say, *"I'll just have a salad,"* and actually mean it.

9.14. Incorporate More Fibre-Rich Foods into Your Diet

Fibre is the dietary underdog that doesn't get the flashy headlines but quietly does all the heavy lifting for your health. It's like the designated driver of carbs: responsible, reliable, and guaranteed to keep things moving.

Fibre is a carb, but not the fun kind your body breaks down for energy. Nope, fibre stubbornly refuses to play along, cruising through your digestive system like it's on a sightseeing tour. It doesn't spike your blood sugar or load up your calorie count, making it the dietary equivalent of a free lunch—except it actually exists.

One of fibre's sneakiest tricks is convincing your stomach you've eaten more than you have. Feel full, eat less, win at life. It's like Jedi mind-tricking your appetite into submission. If you've ever wrestled with portion control or treated "serving size" as a mere suggestion, fibre is here to save you from yourself.

Meet the all-stars of fibre-rich foods:

- **Fruits & Veggies**: Berries, apples, pears, oranges, broccoli, and sweet potatoes—because you deserve a rainbow on your plate.
- **Whole Grains**: Oats, quinoa, brown rice, and whole wheat bread. (Yes, bread can be a hero too.)
- **Legumes**: Beans, lentils, and chickpeas—basically the overachievers of the food world.
- **Nuts & Seeds**: Almonds, chia seeds, and flaxseeds, for when you want fibre with a crunch side.

Fibre isn't just about keeping you full. Its posse of low-calorie, nutrient-rich foods also helps you keep your calorie count in check. And those vitamins, minerals, and antioxidants? They're like bonus perks for choosing Team Fibre.

How to Sneak Fibre into Everything:

- **Breakfast**: Oatmeal with fruit and nuts. It's like dessert, but socially acceptable at 7 a.m.
- **Snacks**: Raw veggies with hummus—because chips are overrated.
- **Lunch**: A whole-grain sandwich—proof that carbs can be good for you.

With a bit of planning, you can hit your fibre goals without even trying that hard. And honestly, who wouldn't want a food that makes you healthier while letting you eat more?

9.15. Incorporate More Fruit into Your Diet

Adding more fruit to your diet is the easiest health upgrade you'll ever make. It's like cheating but without the shame. Packed with vitamins, minerals, antioxidants, and just enough sweetness to make you forget about donuts, fruit is nature's way of saying, *"Here, be healthy and enjoy it."*

Not a fan of guzzling plain water? No problem. Fruits like watermelon, oranges, and grapes double as hydration stations. It's like sneaking water into your body disguised as a snack.

Fresh fruit is the Celebrity Diva of the fruit world: always the best option. But if fresh isn't an option, frozen and canned fruits are solid backups—as long as they haven't been drowned in syrup or sweetened to oblivion. Remember, the closer your fruit is to looking like it fell off a tree, the better it is for you.

- **Breakfast Boost**: Toss some berries on your oatmeal or yogurt. Instant health points unlocked.
- **Snack Attack**: Munch on an apple, banana, or a handful of grapes. No prep, no fuss, just bite and go.
- **Lunch Remix**: Add orange slices or pomegranate seeds to your salad. Yes, fruit in salad is a thing, and yes, it's fantastic.
- **Smooth Operator**: Blend up a smoothie with frozen fruit, a splash of juice, and maybe some spinach if you're feeling extra virtuous.
- **Dessert Upgrade**: Swap cake for a fruit salad. Okay, that's a lie—add fruit to the cake. Half your usual service and replace the other half with a serving of fruit.

Ever had a dragon fruit? A papaya? A passionfruit? Fruits come in more varieties than you can shake a stick at, so get creative. Worst case, you try something new. In the best case, you discover a new obsession.

Incorporating fruit into your day isn't just good for your body; it's also a win for your taste buds. After all, if you're going to eat healthy, it might as well be delicious.

9.16.   Choose Whole Grains

Let's talk grains: the good, the bad, and the fluffy white lies. Spoiler alert—whole grains are the Bruce Wayne of carbs: rich, complex, and way better for you than their bland, over-processed cousins.

Refined grains are like those shady used cars: they look good on the surface but have stripped-out interiors. Bye-bye bran and germ, hello nutrient void. Sure, they're light, fluffy, and comforting, but so is your pillow—and you shouldn't eat that either.

Whole grains keep their bran, germ, and endosperm intact, meaning you get fibre, vitamins, and minerals all in one bite. Benefits? Oh, just minor things like:

- Lower risk of heart disease (because who has time for clogged arteries?)
- Reduced chances of T2DM (sweets are supposed to be occasional, not your diagnosis).
- Keeping certain cancers at bay (because grains are busy doing your bodyguard duties).

And bonus: whole grains are filling. That means fewer snack attacks at 3 p.m. when you start eyeballing vending machine candy bars like a lost lover.

- "100% Whole Grain" or "100% Whole Wheat": The real MVPs.
- "Multi-Grain": Could be whole grains... or could be cardboard painted pretty.
- "Wheat": As vague as a bad Tinder bio.

If the first ingredient isn't "whole," put it back on the shelf like it's on fire.

- **Whole Wheat Bread**: Great for sandwiches, toast, or pretending your avocado obsession is balanced.
- **Oatmeal**: The breakfast staple that says, *"I care about myself today."*
- **Quinoa**: Technically a seed, but we let it hang with the grains because it's a protein-packed overachiever.
- **Brown Rice**: Makes your stir-fry smarter.
- **Whole Grain Pasta**: For when you're carb-loading for... sitting on the couch.

The next time someone tries to serve you plain white bread, remember that life is too short to eat boring carbs. Go whole, or go home.

9.17. Add Beans and Legumes to Your Meals

Beans and legumes might not have the flashy allure of a steak or the Instagram-worthy appeal of avocado toast, but they're your kitchen team's dependable, cost-effective MVPs. Think of them as the hardworking sidekicks of nutrition: not glamorous, but absolutely essential.

1. **Fibre Powerhouses**: Keeping your digestion regular like a Swiss train schedule.
2. **Protein Packed**: Who needs overpriced protein powders when chickpeas have your back?
3. **Low in Fat**: Unlike that "healthy" salad drowning in ranch dressing.
4. **Loaded with Nutrients**: Iron for energy, folate for your blood and brain, and magnesium for chill vibes.

Beans and legumes are like the leftovers that get better with time. Cook them in bulk, freeze them, and you've got an arsenal of nutrition ready for anything. Feeling fancy? Toss them into:

- **Salads**: Because lettuce can't carry the team alone.
- **Soups & Stews**: Warm, comforting, and sneakily healthy.
- **Casseroles**: Because life needs cheesy, beany goodness sometimes.
- **Tacos**: Black beans, meet tortilla. Match made in heaven.

- **Soak 'Em**: Not just for reducing cooking time—this also makes them less, um, musical.
- **Spice It Up**: Beans are the blank canvas of food—throw in garlic, cumin, or paprika to jazz things up.
- **Don't Fear the Canned Aisle**: Rinse off that salty brine, and they're good to go.

Why spend $$$ on fancy cuts of meat when kidney beans are over here being cheap, filling, and eco-friendly? They also don't come with a side of guilt about your carbon footprint.

If you're still turning your nose up at beans, remember this: they're nutritious, sustainable, and make you feel fuller for longer. Plus, who doesn't want to eat something that's saving both your wallet and the planet?

9.18.   Snack on Nuts and Seeds

They may be small, but nuts and seeds pack a punch that even protein bars envy. These miniature powerhouses are the snack equivalent of a Swiss Army knife—versatile, nutritious, and always ready to save the day.

1. **Protein & Fibre**: Your one-two punch against mid-afternoon hunger.
2. **Healthy Fats**: The good kind that says, *"I care about your heart."*
3. **Vitamins & Minerals**: From magnesium to zinc, they've got your back (and bones).
4. **Portable**: The snack you can toss in your bag and forget about until you're starving in traffic.

- **Almonds**: The overachiever of the nut world—good for snacking, baking, and crushing into almond butter or milk.
- **Walnuts**: Brain food, because they look like little brains. Coincidence? I think not.
- **Pistachios**: Built-in portion control thanks to their shells. Unless you're a maniac with a de-shelling technique.
- **Pumpkin Seeds**: Because your Jack-o'-Lantern leftovers shouldn't go to waste.
- **Chia Seeds**: Tiny, but mighty. Add them to yogurt and watch them poof into fibre-rich pudding.

Beware of the portion creep. A handful of almonds? Fantastic. The whole bag in one sitting? Congratulations, you've just consumed the calorie equivalent of a triple cheeseburger. Opt for unsalted, unflavoured options unless you want your heart doing cardio from all that sodium.

- **Solo Snack**: They're like that friend who can handle a party solo. Always a hit.
- **Sprinkle Power**: On salads, yogurt, or oatmeal. Instant upgrade.
- **Blend It**: Toss the seeds into smoothies for a satisfying crunch—or a blender brawl if you forget to soak them.

Nuts and seeds are proof that good things come in small packages. They're delicious, nutritious, and the perfect partner for your snack game. Keep your portions in check unless you're bulking... or trying to become a squirrel's best friend.

9.19. Focus On Quality, Not Quantity

Forget obsessively counting calories—actual health starts with what's on your plate, not just the numbers behind it. Instead of fixating on every crumb, focus on filling your meals with nutrient-packed options that fuel your body and mind.

1. **Nutrient-Dense = More Bang for Your Bite**: Foods rich

in fibre, protein, and healthy fats provide essential nutrients without the crash that comes with empty calories.

2. **Long-Lasting Satisfaction**: Whole, nutritious foods keep you fuller longer, making that 3 p.m. vending machine run a thing of the past.
3. **Sustainable Habits**: It's easier to stick to a diet that feels like a lifestyle, not a punishment.

- **Fruits & Vegetables**: Nature's multivitamins, loaded with antioxidants, fibre, and flavour.
- **Whole Grains**: Think quinoa, oats, and brown rice—not the overly processed white stuff.
- **Healthy Fats**: Avocados, nuts, seeds, and olive oil—because your brain and heart deserve the best.
- **Lean Proteins**: Beans, lentils, fish, and poultry—fuel for muscles and metabolism.

- **Variety is Key**: Rotate your foods to avoid boredom and ensure you're getting a broad spectrum of nutrients.
- **Flavour Boosters**: Spices, herbs, and healthy condiments can turn even the simplest dishes into gourmet experiences.
- **Colour Your Plate**: A rainbow of food isn't just Instagram-worthy—it's a sign of a well-rounded meal.

When you focus on the quality of your food, you build a sustainable eating plan that prioritizes health and enjoyment. No more yo-yo dieting or endless hunger—just a happier, healthier you.

So, the next time you're meal planning, think less about restrictions and more about abundance—an abundance of nutrients, flavours, and vibrant foods that make healthy eating a joy, not a chore.

9.20. Focus on Portion Sizes

Portion control is the unsung villain of your midnight pizza binge. Even if you're inhaling kale smoothies and quinoa bowls, too much of a good thing is still... too much. Those "healthy" calories? Yeah, they'll still pack their bags and take up residence on your thighs if you overdo it.

Every bite you take whispers, *"I'm just a little calorie; I couldn't hurt you!"* But consume more than your body needs, and those calories morph into fat reserves faster than you can say *"second helping."* It's like inviting a charming guest to your house who refuses to leave and starts inviting his friends and changing his mailing address to yours.

- **Measuring Cups and Scales**: Because nothing says *"I'm living my best life"* like weighing your chicken breast to the gram.
- **Portion Size Education**: Learn what a "typical" portion looks like. Spoiler: it's not the entire casserole dish.
- Eyeballing Portions: Eventually, you'll be that person who knows what three ounces of salmon looks like. Party trick? Probably not.

Eating too fast isn't just impolite—it's a ticket to overeating town. Your stomach needs time to notify your brain that it's full. But no, you had to wolf down that burger like wolves were chasing you. Slow down. Savour. Pretend you're on some avant-garde cooking show where every bite must be dramatically appreciated.

You can still have your cake and eat it, too—just not the whole cake. Enjoy that chocolate lava dessert, but treat it like a forbidden lover you meet only on special occasions. Balance it with a sad salad and call it a win.

Portion control isn't about deprivation—it's about making sure you don't become a walking PSA for overindulgence. Embrace the small victories, savour your food, and remember: you're just one bite away from chaos.

9.21. Cut No More Than 10% Of Your Total Calorie Intake

So, you've decided to cut calories. Good for you! But before you go all in and survive on celery sticks and existential dread, remember: slow and steady wins the race—or at least doesn't land you in the hospital. Reduce by just enough, not so much that your body thinks it's auditioning for a survival show.

For example, if your body needs 2,000 calories daily to keep things running smoothly, don't slash it to 1,200 in a misguided attempt to become a calorie martyr. Try 1,800. That's enough to make a difference without turning you into a hangry gremlin.

- **Nutrient Deficiencies**: Those "lose 20 pounds in two weeks" diets come with a side of anemia, brittle bones, and a malfunctioning immune system. Sounds fun, right?
- **Gallstones**: Who knew your gallbladder could have a meltdown over your diet? Spoiler: it can. And gallstone surgery isn't the glow-up you were hoping for.
- **Dehydration**: You might lose "water weight," but congratulations, you're now dizzy, fatigued, and have a headache big enough to double as a horror movie subplot.

Lose weight too fast, and you'll shed muscle along with fat. And muscle isn't just for flexing—it's what keeps your metabolism revving. Less muscle means a slower BMR, which translates to burning fewer calories while doing absolutely nothing. Talk about a bad deal.

Instead of crash dieting, try subtle sabotage:

- Swap out chips for carrots.
- Walk an extra 10 minutes daily.
- Drink water instead of sodas or your daily tears of despair.

This way, you'll reach your goals without alienating your body or sanity. Remember: it's not about losing weight quickly; it's about keeping it off without losing your mind or gallbladder.

9.22.   Set Realistic Goals

Listen, if you're looking for a magic pill or a quick fix to lose pounds faster than a Disney+ movie cancellation, you're in the wrong place. Weight management is about setting goals that are more about *"I'll still be alive and functional"* than *"I want to look like a supermodel by next weekend."*

Aim for no more than 1% of your body weight per week, or 4% per month. Yeah, that's right—no drastic "I'll drop 20 pounds this weekend" kind of plan. It might not seem like much, but those little numbers stack up when you're in it for the long haul (and not some temporary fad). In a few months, you'll be looking at a number that could impress even the gym bros, and you'll still have the energy to, you know, live.

Losing weight slowly gives your body time to adjust. It's like being handed a gadget with no instruction manual and figuring it out one button at a time. When you rush it, it's like smashing all the buttons at once and hoping for the best. You'll probably end up with muscle loss, nutrient deficiencies, or—worst of all—an unhealthy relationship with food. Slow it down, and your body won't revolt by making your metabolism a sloth.

Weight loss isn't the 100-meter dash. You're in it for the long run, so stop treating it like a race to the nearest bakery. Be patient with yourself and remind yourself that Rome wasn't built in a day. Celebrate those little victories (like not face-planting into a bag of cheesecake after a stressful day), and focus on long-term health rather than short-term glory.

Don't stress if you're not losing a pound every week. Instead, focus on making tiny adjustments, like swapping out a soda for water or parking farther away from the store. These little actions will add up over time, and soon, you'll realize that slow and steady really does win the race. Just make sure your body's still functional by the finish line.

In short, set goals that are realistic and sustainable. Don't kill yourself over losing a few pounds in one month. Instead, celebrate the small wins and remember, it's not about how fast you can shed the weight—it's about making changes that stick around longer than that last bag of chips you promised yourself you'd never open.

9.23. Calculate Your Target Weight Loss

Now, let's get the calculator out and do some math. But before you panic and start Googling "how to lose 20 pounds overnight," let's take a realistic approach.

First things first, figure out how much weight you want to lose. It's like planning a road trip: you need a destination. You're not just going to hop in the car and hope you get somewhere, right? Same deal with weight loss. Consider your current weight, body composition (because muscle weighs more than fat, duh), and overall health. Do some math if you're 200 pounds and want to lose 20.

You've got your target weight loss in mind, now apply the golden rule: no more than 1% of your body weight per week. For example, if you're 200 pounds, that's no more than 2 pounds a week. Sure, it won't have you looking like a Hollywood model in a week, but you're being smart about it. Healthy weight loss isn't about fast results; it's about gradual changes that last longer than a cake in front of some of your friends.

Here's the hard truth: weight loss isn't a straight line. You might lose 2 pounds one week, and then the next week, it's just water retention and hormonal chaos throwing off your rhythm. One day, the scale's your best friend; the next day, it's your worst enemy. So don't obsess over the scale like it's a cult leader. Focus on the big picture—healthy habits and consistency.

Instead of racing to the scale's approval, focus on sustainable lifestyle changes. Swap a sugary drink for water, have a salad instead of fries, and move your body in ways that don't feel like punishment. Small, consistent changes over time will help you achieve your weight loss goal without becoming a crazy, hangry version of yourself.

Remember, the goal is to make gradual changes, not drastic ones. If you lose 1 pound a week, that's 4 pounds in a month— congratulations, you're doing great! And if your weight fluctuates, don't lose your mind. Please stick to the plan and let the weight loss happen in its own time. You'll hit your target weight, feel healthier, and maybe even have a few less emotional breakdowns over the scale. Now, that's a win.

9.24. Stay Hydrated with Water as Your Primary Beverage

Staying hydrated is your body's way of saying, **"Hey, don't forget I'm 60% water and not a cactus!"** It's crucial for everything from keeping you cool to ensuring your muscles don't rebel mid-squat. Plus, let's be honest: dehydration turns your brain into a cranky, overheated potato—not ideal when trying to crush your fitness goals.

The first rule of the hydration club is to drink water—a lot of it. Aim for at least 8 cups a day—roughly 2 litres, or 64 ounces, if you're into the fancy measurements. If you're living in a hot climate, hitting the gym, or just sweating through life, bump that up a bit. Your body will thank you by not turning into a raisin.

During exercise, aim for about 250 ml every 20 minutes. You'll probably need more if you're doing intense workouts or pretending to be a triathlete.

Pro tip: Carry a water bottle, preferably one so obnoxiously large it could double as a weapon in self-defence. Not only will it remind you to hydrate, but it'll also make you look serious about your liquid priorities.

Water is like the unsung hero of healthy living—it helps your body function properly, regulates your temperature, transports nutrients, and flushes out toxins. It's the ultimate multitasker. But wait, there's more! Water can even help you feel fuller, which means you might not need that extra bag of chips. Water is, quite literally, a free weight loss ally.

If you think plain water is as exciting as watching paint dry, it's time for a makeover. Toss some lemon, lime, or berries in there for a little zest. Herbal teas and decaf coffee also count toward your daily hydration quota, so feel free to sip away. But don't get fooled into thinking sugary sodas and alcohol are hydration's BFFs. They're not. They'll only dehydrate you and leave you with a bloated belly—and we're not here for that.

Water is simple, effective, and, dare I say, the secret to life. Keep it classy, keep yourself hydrated, and watch your body run like a fully charged EV. So go ahead, raise your glass to the most underrated part of a healthy lifestyle: water.

9.25. Choose Fruit Juices with Reasonable Amounts of Sugar

Let's talk about fruit juice, that supposedly healthy option you reach for when you're feeling fancy—but hold your horses, my friend. Not all juices are created equal. Some can be sneakier than a Canadian goose in a supermarket, packing in the sugars and empty calories while masquerading as healthy.

Sure, fruit juice is better than sugary sodas, but that doesn't mean it's guilt-free. Some juices are loaded with added sugars that'll have you questioning whether you're drinking fruit juice or liquid candy. Choose 100% fruit juice with no added sugars or syrups when scanning labels. It's like the purest form of juice—think of it as the juice of royalty.

It's easy to drink a whole glass of fruit juice in one sitting without realizing how much sugar and calories you've just consumed. Trust me, your body won't thank you later. So, here's the plan: try diluting your juice with water, or opt for smaller serving sizes. You'll still get that fruity fix, but with fewer sugar crashes.

Here's the kicker—fruit juice can't replace the real deal. Whole fruits are packed with fibre, which helps with digestion and keeps you feeling full. So, if you're all about that juice life, consider pairing it with a piece of whole fruit for the ultimate nutrient combo. And if you're already doing the healthy thing with juice, make sure it's just one part of your balanced diet that includes plenty of whole foods.

Fruit juice can be a solid choice in moderation, but don't let it trick you into thinking it's the magical health potion of the century. Be savvy, watch your portions, and keep the sugar intake in check. That way, you can sip with confidence, knowing you're making the best choice for your body.

9.26. Avoid Dehydrating Agents Like Coffee and Alcohol

Hydration is the thing we all know we should do, but we sometimes forget it until we're parched and our tongues stick to the roof of our mouths. Staying hydrated throughout the day is critical, but the drinks you choose can make all the difference. While that cup of coffee or glass of wine might sound appealing, let's break down their potential to sabotage your hydration efforts.

We all know coffee is that morning magic potion, but too much of it can be a dehydrating culprit. Caffeine, that lovely thing that gives us life, is a natural diuretic. This means it makes you pee more than you might like, leading to dehydration if you're not careful. So go ahead, enjoy your daily cup of joe—but let's stick to less of it and make sure you're sipping water alongside it. Hydration and caffeine? A win-win.

We all love a glass of wine or a cold beer now and then (or maybe a little more often), but here's the catch: alcohol doesn't help with hydration. In fact, it has a lovely little dehydrating effect on your body. Alcohol increases urine production, meaning you could end up losing more fluid than you're taking in. So, if you're hitting the bar or drinking at home, remember to balance it with some water. Your body will thank you by keeping a hangover at bay the next day.

When it comes to caffeine and alcohol, moderation is key. Keep your coffee to one cup and alcohol to one drink for women and two for men (unless you're looking for a party—then I don't judge, but please hydrate). Between your beverages of choice, make sure water is your trusty sidekick. Your body will be happier, and you'll avoid the dreaded dehydration hangover (whether it's from caffeine or alcohol).

Coffee, alcohol, and the rest of your favourite beverages are fine in moderation as long as you're mindful of how they affect your hydration levels. So, enjoy your cup of coffee or glass of wine, but remember to drink water and keep your hydration game strong. After all, water is the true hero of your wellness story.

9.27. Eat Hydrating Foods

We all know water is the top contender when it comes to hydration, but did you know that certain foods are also packed with water to keep you refreshed and nourished throughout the day? That's right, hydration isn't just about what you drink—it's also about what you eat.

First up, let's talk about watermelon, the fruit that's basically the water bottle of the fruit world. With a whopping 92% water content, watermelon doesn't just quench your thirst—it practically bathes you in hydration. If you're craving something fresh and juicy, watermelon is your hero.

Next, there's cucumbers—who knew this crunchy veggie was so hydrating? With about 95% water, cucumbers are perfect for snacking, tossing into salads, or adding to your water for a fun twist.

Let's not forget berries—strawberries, raspberries, blueberries—whatever your favourites may be. These little antioxidant-packed gems are delicious and offer a healthy dose of water. Toss them in yogurt, snack on them by the handful, or add them to your smoothie for an extra hydrating punch.

Now, let's talk about leafy greens like lettuce, spinach, and kale. These veggies are filled with essential nutrients and high in water. Imagine getting your vitamins and hydration all in one bite! Throw these into your salads, wraps, or even your morning smoothie for a green, water-packed boost to your day.

Incorporating more water-rich fruits and vegetables into your meals allows you to stay hydrated without constantly reaching for a glass. Watermelon, cucumbers, berries, and leafy greens are your new hydration squad—ready to help you keep your fluid levels up and your body feeling fresh. So, the next time you're feeling thirsty, remember: a snack might just do the trick!

9.28.   Focus on Balance

Let's face it: extreme diets that eliminate entire food groups are a thing of the past. The key to maintaining health and hitting your weight goals isn't about cutting things out but balance and variety. That means enjoying a wide range of nutrient-packed foods that nourish your body without making yourself feel deprived.

First, fruits and vegetables should take up a big chunk of your plate. These little wonders are packed with fibre, vitamins, and minerals—and they're low in calories. Leafy greens, berries, citrus fruits, bell peppers, and squash are perfect for a colourful, nutrient-rich diet. Plus, the more colour on your plate, the better for your health (and your Facebook posts).

Remember, don't skip out on whole grains like brown rice, quinoa, and whole wheat bread. They're more than just a side dish—they're an excellent source of fibre and essential nutrients. Whole grains help keep your digestion in check, stabilize blood sugar, and keep you feeling fuller for longer. Just try not to eat an entire loaf of whole-wheat bread. Moderation is key!

Protein is crucial for building and repairing tissues, so ensure you get your fill. Chicken, fish, and legumes like beans and lentils are all fantastic choices that provide the essential amino acids your body craves. Whether you prefer a juicy piece of grilled chicken or a hearty serving of lentils, lean proteins will make you feel satisfied and strong.

Finally, let's talk about healthy fats. Sounds like an oxymoron, right? But trust me, nuts, seeds, and avocados are the good fat that helps maintain your health while keeping you feeling full. They also provide essential fatty acids that support your brain, heart, and overall well-being. So go ahead, add some guac to your salad—your body will thank you.

Achieving your weight goals isn't about banning entire food groups—it's about creating a balanced and varied diet that fuels your body with everything it needs. You'll feel great and keep your body running smoothly with a mix of fruits, veggies, whole grains, lean proteins, and healthy fats. Just remember: moderation, variety, and balance are your best friends on this journey. So go ahead and load up that plate—your health will thank you.

9.29. Be on a Diet That You Can Turn into a Lifestyle

Let's face it: the quick-fix diets that promise rapid weight loss often lead to disappointment and frustration. You start with enthusiasm, only to find that the strict rules or food restrictions are hard to maintain in the long run. If you're looking for lasting results, the secret lies in finding a diet that works with your lifestyle and can be sustained over time.

Instead of choosing restrictive diets that ban entire food groups or demand unwavering discipline, why not opt for a balanced approach? A nutrient-dense diet that includes fruits, vegetables, whole grains, lean proteins, and healthy fats offers more flexibility and variety. This kind of eating plan is not just a short-term fix but a sustainable way to promote overall health and manage weight in the long run.

Let's be honest: if you don't like the foods in your diet plan, you won't stick with it. Enjoyment is a critical factor in the success of any diet. The key is to choose a way of eating that aligns with your preferences. Look for foods you love, and explore creative recipes and new cooking techniques to make healthy eating fun and satisfying. You're more likely to maintain a diet if it includes meals you look forward to eating.

Weight loss isn't just about what you eat—it's about how much and how often. Mindful eating and portion control are essential to avoid overeating, even with healthy foods. Pay attention to your body's hunger and fullness cues, and be conscious of your overall calorie intake. This will allow you to balance enjoying your meals and achieving your weight management goals.

The ultimate goal is to turn healthy eating into a lifestyle, not a temporary diet. By choosing a sustainable eating plan that you can enjoy, experiment with, and maintain, you're setting yourself up for long-term success. With a balanced diet that aligns with your goals and supports your overall health, you can achieve the lifestyle change you've been looking for.

9.30.   Do Not Skip Meals

Skipping meals might seem like the shortcut to caloric glory, but here is a plot twist: your body doesn't care about your half-baked plan. Instead, it kicks into survival mode faster than you can say "intermittent fasting." By dinner, your inner gremlin takes over, and suddenly, you're devouring a 6-person family meal, a pint of ice cream, and possibly a sleeve of cookies for good measure. Nice job—you've officially out-eaten the meal you skipped, which probably angered your pancreas in the process.

But wait, it gets better. Your metabolism? Yeah, it's filing for early retirement. Skipping meals signals to your body, *"Hey, famine's here!"* So, instead of burning calories like a functioning organism, your metabolism decides to chill harder than a sloth in a hammock. Congrats, you're now losing weight at the pace of evolution.

And while you're out there living the no-meal dream, your body's quietly falling apart. No breakfast? Great, now you're low on iron and calcium. Skipped lunch? Say hello to brittle bones and vitamin D deficiency. But hey, scurvy's totally retro, right? Who needs a functioning immune system when you can save a whopping 300 calories?

Here's a radical idea: eat your meals. Crazy, I know. It doesn't need to be a five-star feast—just real food that won't leave you feral by 9 p.m. Throw in some fruits, veggies, lean protein, and maybe a grain or two. Not only will your body thank you, but you'll also stop raiding the pantry like a raccoon at midnight. It's a win-win.

9.31. Do Not Deprive Yourself

Let's get one thing clear: healthy eating doesn't mean becoming some soulless kale-chomping machine who winces at the sight of a cupcake. No, life's too short for that kind of misery. You can have your cake and eat it too—just don't propose to it and make it the centre of your universe.

Here's the deal: moderation is key. If you ban yourself from all the good stuff, your brain will inevitably stage a rebellion, screaming,

"Cookies! Now!" And before you know it, you've blacked out, only to wake up surrounded by empty cookie wrappers, sticky fingers, and shame. A lot of soldiers have fallen like this.

Instead of swinging between complete denial and unhinged gluttony, try this wild concept: balance. Sure, have that slice of pizza, but maybe don't wash it down with a milkshake the size of your head. Toss some veggies into the mix. I know they're not the exciting part of the meal, but hey, they're what keep your insides from staging a revolt.

Healthy eating isn't a joyless punishment—it's about building habits that let you eat the occasional donut without having a full existential crisis. So, eat the cake. Just don't elope with it. We both know it's a toxic relationship.

9.32. Incorporate Physical Activity

The magical cure-all that somehow makes you feel like you're both conquering the world and questioning your life choices at the same time. Let's talk about how it can help you not just with weight loss but with, you know, staying alive. Seriously, regular physical activity can lower your risk of developing heart disease, T2DM, and even certain cancers. So, there's that—nothing too dramatic.

Now, the American Heart Association says we should aim for at least 150 minutes of moderate-intensity aerobic activity or 75 minutes of vigorous-intensity exercise a week. Yeah, that sounds like a lot, but I'm not asking you to run a marathon here. Moderate stuff includes brisk walking, cycling, or even swimming—activities that make you feel like you've done something without needing a nap afterward. On the other hand, if you're feeling wild, try some vigorous exercise—running, jumping rope, or maybe a basketball game where you almost die of exhaustion but still call it "fun."

Let's not forget strength training. It's not just for bodybuilders or those who want to look like they've been chiselled from stone. Lifting weights (or doing bodyweight exercises) boosts your metabolism, which means you're burning calories even while binge-watching Crave TV. Aim for at least two strength training sessions a week. Your muscles will thank you—or at least, they'll hurt in the morning as a reminder of your effort.

The key here is to find something you enjoy—yes, that's right. Exercise doesn't have to be a punishment. So, pick something that doesn't make you feel like you're being tortured by a medieval trainer, and make it a regular habit. Then watch as your weight management journey becomes a little less painful and a little more fun.

9.33.   Start With a Warm-Up

Everyone's least favourite part of working out. It's the necessary evil you know you should do but somehow always want to skip because, let's face it, the treadmill is calling your name, and it's so much easier to dive straight into the "good stuff." But here's the deal: skipping your warm-up is like driving a car without warming up the engine first. You can do it, but things might not go so smoothly.

A proper warm-up gets your heart pumping, warms up your muscles, and prepares your body for the torture you're about to put it through. Plus, it helps you avoid those oh-so-dramatic injuries that make you feel like you're starring in your own personal tragedy.

Start with some light cardio—nothing fancy, just enough to get the blood flowing and your heart rate up. Jogging in place or brisk walking for about 5-10 minutes should do the trick. It's time for dynamic stretches once your body's a little warmer. And no, this isn't a fancy term for random flailing. These stretches involve movement and help activate the muscles you're about to use. Think walking lunges, high knees, butt kicks (yes, you'll look ridiculous, but it's worth it), and arm circles.

You can also sneak in some bodyweight exercises, like squats or push-ups, to warm up even more. The goal is to get your muscles ready to work without putting them in a chokehold right away.

So, before you dive into your workout like a kid on Christmas morning, take a few minutes to warm up. Your muscles (and your ego) will thank you when you're not hobbling off the treadmill in agony later.

9.34.   Focus on Full-Body Stretches

Stretching is not just about touching your toes with your fingers in a desperate bid for flexibility. If you want to avoid pulling a muscle and possibly creating a YouTube-worthy fail, you must stretch your whole body, not just those stiff shoulders or hamstrings that have been crying out for attention.

Think of your body as a complicated machine with many moving parts—neck, shoulders, arms, wrists, back, hips, legs, and ankles. If one part of that machine is out of whack, it could throw off your entire performance. So, make sure to stretch everything. When you stretch all these areas, you're not just improving flexibility and range of motion but also reducing the chances of injury while you work out like a fitness guru in training.

Start with basic full-body stretches, such as standing quad stretches (yes, the one where you grab your ankle and try not to faceplant), seated forward folds (bend, but don't snap), downward-facing dog (not as easy as it looks, but so worth it), and spinal twists (a great way to pretend you're a contortionist).

Yoga poses are a nice touch, too—try the warrior (for that *"I'm in control"* vibe), tree (perfect for days when you feel like you're about to fall apart), or pigeon (because stretching your hips makes you feel like a serene yogi).

The key? Don't be that person forcing their body into positions it clearly doesn't want to go. Stretch gently and gradually, and listen to your body—it will let you know when you're overdoing it. You don't need to go full circus contortionist; just a few moments of controlled stretching to help you stay injury-free.

9.35. Hold Each Stretch for at Least 30 Seconds

Stretching isn't just about posing like a gymnast for 5 seconds and calling it a day. If you really want to make those muscles stretch like you're auditioning for The Flex Factor, you need to hold each stretch for at least 30 seconds. That's right, 30 seconds is the magic number. Research has shown that the longer you hold a stretch, the better it helps lengthen muscle fibres and boosts elasticity. So, patience is key if you're trying to be as flexible as a rubber band.

Now, when you stretch, don't go full: *"I'm going to touch my toes even if it kills me."* You want to feel tension in the muscle—yes, tension, but not pain. If it hurts, you've gone too far, my friend, and that's just a one-way ticket to injury town. So, stop before it becomes a full-on muscle scream.

And here's a pro tip: breathe. Deeply, slowly, like you're meditating or trying to calm down after seeing your phone bill. The more relaxed you are, the better the stretch will work its magic.

Stretching isn't just a fancy way to look like you know what you're doing in the gym. It's also great for reducing muscle soreness and improving circulation. So, give your muscles the love they deserve by holding those stretches long enough to actually do something— and get ready to feel like a yoga master who's got all the flexibility in the world.

9.36. Make Stretching a Habit

You gotta make it a part of your daily routine without feeling like you're trying to add another chore to your list. Sure, committing to it takes a little effort—like anything worth doing—but once you get into the groove, it'll feel like second nature. Just set aside specific times each day to stretch. You know, like before or after your workout, or even during that 3 p.m. slump at work when you're trying not to faceplant into your keyboard.

The key to sticking with it is making it something you actually want to do, not something that feels like a punishment. So, add some relaxing music, light a candle (if you're into that whole zen vibe), or find a stretching buddy who'll remind you to stop being a couch potato. Find a good rhythm and environment, and soon enough, stretching will become something you look forward to instead of avoiding, like your last-minute gym membership.

And remember: when stretching becomes a habit, you're not just improving flexibility. You're building a routine that your body will thank you for every single day.

9.37. Set Achievable Goals

Setting goals is like setting a GPS for your fitness journey— without them, you might end up driving in circles or, worse, stuck in a never-ending loop of *"I'll start tomorrow."* The trick is to keep things realistic and not aim for impossible feats like *"I'll lose 20 pounds in a week"* (unless you've found a magical diet secret that no one else knows about, and in that case, please share). Instead, break it down: aim to lose 1 pound per week, or maybe add a few more minutes to your workout time each week. Small wins lead to big victories.

Get specific with your goals! Instead of saying, *"I'll work out more,"* try, *"I'll work out for 30 minutes, four times a week,"* and work from there. It's important to start where you are, so if your current fitness level is more couch potato than marathon runner, give yourself some grace. Ease into it with shorter workouts, and slowly level up. Rome wasn't built in a day, and neither are six-pack abs (unless you're one of those people, and again, please share your secrets).

Tracking your progress is essential—think of it as checking your map to see how far you've come. If you're into that vintage vibe, you can use fitness apps, trackers, or just the trusty pen-and-paper method. The key is consistency. Progress might be slow at first, but trust the process. When you look back and see how far you've come, those setbacks will seem like tiny bumps in the road, not the end of the world.

So, be patient, celebrate the little wins, and remember that fitness is a marathon, not a sprint—unless you're running a marathon, in which case, good for you!

9.38. Incorporate Cardio Exercise into Your Routine

Cardio exercise is like your body's personal health superhero—it helps you burn calories, boosts endurance, and gives your heart some well-deserved TLC. If you don't get your heart rate up for at least 150 minutes of moderate cardio or 75 minutes of intense cardio a week, you're missing out on that sweet, sweet cardiovascular goodness.

The great thing about cardio is that it doesn't have to be a "one size fits all" activity. You can go for a run, bike like you're in the Tour de France, or make a splash with some swimming. If you're more of an indoor workout kind of person, the elliptical machine, stair stepper, or cycling can give you that cardio fix without the sunburn. Bonus: everyday activities count, too—take the stairs instead of the elevator or take a brisk walk at lunch to add some sneaky cardio to your day.

Starting slow is your best friend here—no need to sprint out of the gate and burn out in the first week. Ease into it, listen to your body (it's probably begging for a break at some point), and slowly increase your workout duration and intensity. There's no medal for overdoing it, so give yourself grace and remember that consistency is the key. You got this!

9.39.   Incorporate Strength Training

Strength training is like giving your muscles a VIP pass to the calorie-burning party. Building muscle doesn't just make you look more muscular; it cranks up your BMR, which means you burn more calories even when you're doomscrolling YouTube shorts. So, what's not to love?

Focus on exercises that work multiple muscle groups for maximum impact. Squats, lunges, push-ups, and rows are all solid choices. They're like the all-you-can-eat buffet of strength training—working your legs, core, and upper body at the same time. Plus, you don't need a fancy gym to get in on the action. Bodyweight exercises, like planks, mountain climbers, and burpees, can turn your living room into a personal gym. Get creative with household items—bags of flour, heavy books, or even your dog (if your dog's cool with it) can work as weights.

Start with a weight that's right for you—don't go from zero to Hercules in one session. Gradually increase the weight as you get stronger, but always make sure to give yourself at least one rest day between sessions to let your muscles recover. As you get stronger, you can amp up the intensity and length of your strength sessions, ensuring your muscles never get bored. Get ready to lift your way to a stronger you!

9.40.   Monitor Your Progress

Tracking your progress is like keeping score in a game—without it, you're just guessing if you're winning or not. Whether you're aiming for weight loss, strength, or overall health, there are plenty of ways to see how you're doing.

First up is the workout log. It's your personal scoreboard. It'll show you how much stronger you're getting, how much endurance you've built, and how many calories you've burned. If that's not enough, add a fitness tracker or app to track every step, squat, and calorie. You'll be tracking so much that you'll start to feel like a walking data set.

Now, let's talk numbers: weight and waist circumference. Yes, your weight is a helpful starting point, but it's like checking your blood pressure every five minutes—it fluctuates constantly. So, please don't freak out when it bounces up after a salty dinner. Track your weight over time to spot trends, not fluctuations. For a clearer picture, take a measuring tape to your waist. It's a great way to see where the fat's packing up, and it might give you more accurate feedback on your progress than the dreaded scale ever will.

Lastly, remember that this is a marathon, not a sprint. Celebrate those small wins, like finally getting through your workout without feeling like you're about to die or noticing that your favourite jeans are a little looser. Even if things are moving slowly, stay consistent and trust the process—results are coming, one step at a time.

9.41. Alternate Between High and Low-Volume Training

If your workout routine has been stuck in a rut and you're not seeing results, it might be time to shake things up with periodization. Basically, it's like hitting the refresh button on your workout—because who doesn't love a good change of pace?

One effective way to mix things up is by alternating between high and low-volume training. Here's the deal: high-volume training is when you go lighter on the weights but crank up the reps. It's like your muscles' version of a cardio workout, focusing on endurance and toning. Conversely, low-volume training is all about the heavyweights and fewer reps—think building strength and power. It's like the Hulk version of your workout.

Switching between these two approaches will give your muscles a variety of challenges so they don't get bored (and neither do you). For example, you could do high-volume training for your upper body for one week and then hit the lower body with some low-volume training the next. Talk about keeping your muscles on their toes!

Of course, periodization is not a one-size-fits-all solution. Tailor it to your goals and fitness level, and maybe have a chat with a trainer or coach before you go full throttle with a new routine. They'll help you avoid any workout disasters—trust me.

9.42.   Find an Activity You Enjoy

Finding an activity you enjoy is the key to making that full-body workout a regular thing—because, let's be honest, if it feels like a punishment, you'll skip it faster than you can say, *"I'll start next Monday."* The trick is to find something that doesn't make you want to cry or leave you questioning your life choices.

If you're the outdoorsy type who is convinced nature is the answer to all your problems, hiking, swimming, or kayaking could be your thing. These activities get your whole body moving while letting you pretend that the fresh air and beautiful scenery are enough to drown out the existential dread.

Maybe you prefer a more "social" approach to misery? Try a local fitness class or boot camp. They'll help you meet people, which is nice, but more importantly, they'll keep you motivated to keep up with everyone else, even if it's just so you don't look like a failure in front of strangers.

On the gentler side of things, there's always yoga and Pilates. They stretch and strengthen your muscles, relieve stress, and can help you pretend you're all zen, even though your inner monologue is screaming. Plus, they're low-impact, so you can start slow and still avoid embarrassing yourself in front of the mirror.

For those who crave intensity (or just want a reason to collapse in a heap afterward), High-Intensity Interval Training (HIIT) might be your nightmare come true. Short bursts of soul-crushing exercise followed by brief moments of rest are perfect for burning calories and feeling like you might die, all in under an hour.

Ultimately, the key to sticking with any workout is to experiment until you find something you can't completely hate. When you look forward to it, you're more likely to make it a regular thing—and we both know you need that.

9.43. Take at Least One Day Off per Week

Rest and recovery are like the unsung heroes of fitness—the chill sidekicks that keep you from turning into a broken-down zombie. Sure, pushing yourself in the gym is great, but taking at least one day off a week is non-negotiable. It's the day your body screams, *"Finally, a break!"* and you get to recharge before your muscles file a formal complaint.

Your rest day doesn't mean morphing into a couch-dwelling hermit binge-watching shows until your eyeballs dry out. Light activities like stretching, walking, or yoga are fair game—just don't go all-out as if you're auditioning for Gladiators. Save the heroics for another day.

And hey, if you're dragging yourself around like an extra in a zombie apocalypse, maybe your body's trying to tell you something: *"We need a longer break, buddy."* Muscle soreness and fatigue? Take an extra rest day (or two). No one will revoke your fitness card for being kind to yourself.

But let's get one thing straight—rest days aren't a hall pass to demolish three pizzas and guzzle sodas like it's your last day on Earth. Stick to your healthy habits, maybe indulge in some self-care, like a bath, reading, or hanging out with people who don't judge your workout playlist.

The bottom line is that the rest isn't slacking—it's strategy. Take care of your body so it doesn't revolt, and you'll be stronger, healthier, and way less likely to need an injury pity party.

9.44.   Stay Consistent with Your Workouts

Consistency is the secret sauce to smashing your weight management goals—well, that and maybe not treating cake like one of the major food groups. While rest and recovery are essential (we covered that), your workouts need to show up in your life like that one overly clingy friend who won't take the hint. Aim for at least three workouts a week, and stick to a schedule that works for you—morning, afternoon, or when-you're-not-too-existentially-exhausted o'clock.

Now, let's be real: life happens. You've got meetings, errands, and maybe a mild addiction to scrolling social media. So, instead of stress-sobbing over your packed calendar, fit in mini workouts—like a brisk walk during lunch or a quick 10-minute session of desperately-dancing-to-burn-calories at home. Pro tip: nobody can judge you if they don't see it.

Consistency doesn't mean being perfect—it means showing up and trying, even if that "trying" is a hilariously clumsy plank at 7 p.m. Progress beats perfection every time. So, keep moving, keep trying, and remember: fitness is about commitment, not a flawless Instagram highlight reel.

9.45.   Increase Your Protein Intake When Building Muscle

When building muscle, protein is your best friend—your swole mate, if you will. Think of it as the scaffolding for your gains, made up of amino acids that repair and grow muscle tissue after workouts. Without enough of it, your muscles will throw a tantrum and refuse to grow. So, be sure to sneak protein into every meal and snack like a fitness-savvy ninja.

For protein sources, you've got options. Lean meats and poultry? Classics. Chicken and turkey are the darlings of the gym crowd for a reason. Fish? Not just for fancy dinners—it's packed with protein and omega-3s for overall health. Eggs? The little powerhouses of nutrition (and drama, if you accidentally crack one). Veggies and vegans, don't panic—you've got beans, nuts, seeds, and soy products like tofu and tempeh in your corner. They'll bulk you up without breaking your plant-based vows.

But before you go full protein bro, remember: too much of a good thing can backfire. Overloading on protein might annoy your kidneys or mess with your bones. Stick to about 0.8 grams of protein per kilogram of body weight daily, or a smidge more if you're chasing those muscle gains. Not sure how much you need? That's where healthcare pros come in. They'll guide you without rolling their eyes at your chicken-and-rice obsession.

And here's a plot twist: if you've got kidney issues or other health concerns, the protein party might need to chill. High intake can stress your kidneys, so get a dietitian or doctor in your corner to tailor your protein plan. They'll help you dodge the health pitfalls and keep you lifting heavy without regrets.

So, protein is your ally, whether you're here for the abs, the strength, or just the satisfaction of not getting winded climbing stairs. But like any good ally, use it wisely—and don't forget to call in the experts when needed.

9.46. Work Out in the Morning

Morning workouts are like coffee—but with fewer jitters and more sweat. They're the ultimate metabolism wake-up call, revving your calorie-burning engine and making you feel like a productivity superhero by 9 a.m. Who doesn't want to tackle their to-do list with the energy of someone who just won a treadmill race?

If you're new to the fitness game, morning workouts are also a sneaky way to trick yourself into being consistent. Start your day by sweating it out, and suddenly, you've got a routine that screams *"responsible adult."* Plus, once it's done, you can spend the rest of your day smugly thinking, *"Yeah, I worked out this morning. What did you do?"*

But here's the kicker: not everyone is built for the sunrise sweat fest. If dragging yourself out of bed at dawn feels like cruel and unusual punishment, don't force it. You're not a robot programmed to jog at 6 a.m. Try different times and figure out when your inner beast mode activates—whether it's morning, lunchtime, or the middle of the night. The key is to find a routine that feels more like a personal victory and less like torture.

Bottom line? Exercise is like pizza—it's great no matter when you have it. Just make sure it fits into your life in a way that keeps you coming back for more. Now, go seize the day (or maybe just the dumbbells).

9.47.   Find a Workout Buddy or Group

Working out solo is fine, but let's face it—sometimes you need someone to sympathize with when your arms feel like spaghetti. Enter the workout buddy or fitness group, your built-in hype squad and accountability crew. Plus, misery loves company, right?

Finding a workout partner is like dating but without the awkward first-date small talk. Reach out to friends, family, or even that coworker who won't stop talking about CrossFit. If that fails, the internet's got your back—fitness groups on social media are basically matchmaking services for sweaty people with shared goals.

Here's the magic of a workout buddy: they'll push you to do that extra rep, cheer you on when you finally master burpees (ugh), and shame you into showing up when you'd rather Netflix and snack. Plus, you can laugh at each other's gym fails—like when you totally misjudge the treadmill speed and do an accidental Matrix move.

Groups, on the other hand, are like fitness cults—minus the creepy robes. Whether it's a running club, yoga class, or boot camp, the camaraderie makes you forget your legs are on fire. And who knows, you might even make a friend who shares your love for post-workout pancakes.

Just pick your people wisely. You don't want a workout buddy who cancels more often than they show up or a group that makes you feel like the slowest gazelle in the herd. Find someone or something that matches your energy, and suddenly, sweating it out doesn't seem so bad. Teamwork makes the dream work—or at least makes the burpees less soul-crushing.

9.48.   Join a Gym or a Fitness Class

Joining a gym or fitness class can add excitement and structure to your fitness journey, and let's be real; sometimes, you need a change of scenery from your living room yoga mat. Gyms offer everything from treadmills to free weights, so whether you're a cardio fanatic or an aspiring bodybuilder, you'll have all the tools at your disposal.

If you're the type who thrives in a social setting, group fitness classes could be your jam. Picture yourself in Zumba, vibing to the beat or challenging your limits in a spin class with an instructor who somehow screams louder than a woman in labour. Prefer working solo? A gym with a wide range of equipment lets you customize your workout without judgment (except maybe from that guy who always hogs the bench press).

Here's the trick: pick a gym or class that matches your vibe and your goals. Want one-on-one guidance? Personal trainers can be a game-changer. On a budget? Many gyms offer free trials—think of them as test-driving your future sweat sanctuary. And yes, location matters. If your gym's an hour away, Paramount+ will probably win more often than not.

Most importantly, stay consistent. Lock in a schedule and show up—even on the days when motivation is as absent as your desire to do burpees. Switch up your routine when needed; new workouts keep things fresh and your muscles guessing.

With the right mindset and a gym that fits your lifestyle, you'll reach your goals and maybe even enjoy the journey. Who knows? You might become that person who actually looks forward to leg day. (Hey, it could happen.)

9.49.   Hire a Personal Trainer

If you're new to exercise or have no clue what you're doing (don't worry, we've all been there), hiring a personal trainer might be your golden ticket—or at least your overpriced lottery scratcher. Think of a trainer as your fitness babysitter: they'll hold your hand, cheer you on, and shame you (just a little) when you skip leg day for the third week in a row.

A good personal trainer can help you set "realistic" goals—like not blacking out during a 5-minute warm-up—and tailor a workout plan that fits your unique needs, preferences, and aversion to sweating. They'll also make sure you don't accidentally decapitate yourself with a barbell while trying to impress strangers in the weight room.

And hey, they're not just there to bark orders like a drill sergeant. A trainer can tweak your routine as you progress—because doing the same three exercises forever is only fun if you enjoy the sweet embrace of monotony—and they'll keep you accountable, which is a polite way of saying they'll guilt-trip you into showing up.

Finding a trainer is like dating, except they're actually paid to care about you. Ask your friends, scour the internet, or creepily stalk gyms for someone who looks competent. Just make sure to check their reviews and credentials. You don't want to end up with a trainer who thinks bicep curls are a complete workout plan.

Yes, personal trainers can be pricey, but so is therapy and bariatric surgery. At least with a trainer you'll get shredded abs (or at least the hope of them). Plus, there's something oddly comforting about paying someone to yell at you while you reconsider every life choice that led you to this point.

9.50. Do Not Be Afraid to Ask for Help

Feeling overwhelmed or stuck during your weight loss journey? Don't worry—it's a rite of passage, like accidentally eating an entire pizza while watching "just one more" episode of The Office. The good news? Asking for help is a sign of strength (and sometimes desperation, but let's go with strength). Whether it's from a friend, family member, or healthcare professional, support is the cheat code for levelling up your weight loss game.

If you're battling the scale and losing (ironically), a healthcare professional can swoop in like the nerdy superhero you didn't know you needed. They'll hit you with personalized nutrition, exercise, and weight management advice—none of that "just eat less and move more" nonsense. Plus, they'll monitor your progress, making you less likely to give up when you plateau harder than an aging pop star.

Asking for help doesn't make you weak; it makes you human. And while humans aren't perfect, we are pretty good at teaming up to tackle big problems—like that leftover cake in the fridge or the mystery of where your abs went.

9.51. Celebrate Your Progress

Celebrating your accomplishments on your journey to better health is essential—because if you don't, who will? Your cat? Probably not. Acknowledge the blood, sweat, and tears (hopefully not too much blood) you've poured into this endeavour. Whether it's dropping a few pounds, surviving kale smoothies, or showing up to the gym even when your bed was serenading you, every win deserves a moment of glory.

Treat yourself! No, not with an entire cheesecake—but how about a new pair of sneakers or that overpriced latte everyone raves about? Or, go for a massage to remind your aching muscles that you do appreciate them. And don't forget to brag to your loved ones—because their job is to clap for you, even if they secretly want to keep the chips on the table.

Pro tip: document your progress with photos or measurements. Later, when you're feeling blah, you can look back and marvel at how far you've come—and maybe cringe at those "before" angles.

Remember, it's not about hitting a magic number on the scale. It's about building a life where you feel good, look good, and maybe even run up the stairs without gasping like an asthmatic walrus. So, celebrate every step, and keep crushing it—one kale leaf and gym selfie at a time.

9.52.   Stay Positive

Staying positive during your weight management journey is like trying to keep your cool in traffic—it's tough, but it's necessary. Setbacks will happen. Maybe you ate an entire pizza on a stressful Tuesday. Who hasn't? Instead of spiralling into self-pity, channel your inner motivational coach and shout, *"This is just a plot twist!"*

The key? Realistic goals. Don't aim to look like a fitness influencer by next month (they probably don't even look like that on Tuesday mornings). Break it down: lose a pound, run an extra minute, or survive one spin class without cursing. Each milestone deserves a mini celebration, preferably without cake.

Also, let's talk about self-compassion. You're not a machine. You're a gloriously flawed human who sometimes mistakes cookies for coping mechanisms. Be kind to yourself. Talk to yourself the way you'd talk to a friend—not like a toxic friend, but the good kind who reminds you that Rome wasn't built in a day, and neither is your dream body.

And ditch the obsession with the scale. That smug little number doesn't define you. Focus on the wins that matter: more energy, fewer mid-afternoon crashes, and not gasping for air after two flights of stairs. Those are the real victories—celebrate them with flair (or a nap; naps are good).

Weight management is like assembling IKEA furniture—frustrating, full of setbacks, and sometimes you want to throw the instructions out the window. But, much like that lopsided bookcase, progress is still progress.

Setbacks? They're inevitable. Maybe you devoured a whole cake because your boss sent one too many emails, or your "quick snack" turned into an all-you-can-eat buffet. It happens. Instead of crying over spilled frosting, look at how far you've come. Did you swap that daily soda for water? Take the stairs without cursing gravity? Those wins matter!

Remember, this isn't a fast-food drive-thru where results show up instantly. It's more like a slow-cooker recipe—deliciously worth it, but painfully slow. If you hit a rough patch, don't hit the self-destruct button. Take a breath, recalibrate, and jump back in. One slip-up doesn't undo all your hard work, unless that slip-up involved a trampoline and donuts, in which case... impressive.

Be patient, even if it feels like your patience is thinner than the ice cream you're trying to avoid. Results take time. Celebrate the small stuff—like not eating your feelings for one day. And don't beat yourself up; life's hard enough without you being your own worst critic. Channel your inner cheerleader and keep going. You'll get there, one victory (and occasional donut) at a time.

9.53. Do Not Compare Yourself to Others

Falling into the comparison trap is like trying to win a staring contest with a cat on the internet—you'll always lose, and you'll never understand why. Social media makes it worse, showcasing everyone's "perfect" weight management journey. But let's be real: for every gym selfie, there's an off-screen pizza binge.

Everyone's path is unique. Comparing yourself to someone else is like comparing apples to...pineapples. Sure, they're both "apples," but they're wildly different. Focus on your wins. Did you walk an extra five minutes instead of contemplating the mysteries of the couch cushion? Celebrate that!

If the comparison monster starts creeping in, whip out a journal. Track your progress and write down every small victory. Your journey isn't just about the number on the scale—it's about feeling stronger, happier, and less like you need to fight your jeans every morning.

And flexibility? It's not just for yoga. If something isn't working, ditch it faster than you'd ditch a bad first date. Hate running? Don't run! Try dancing, biking, or pretending you're in an action movie during your workout. Meal plans giving you nightmares? Swap them out for something that doesn't feel like a punishment.

Above all, remember this: your journey is yours. Everyone else can have their kale smoothies and CrossFit cults. You're here for what works for you. So, grab that apple, stay adaptable, and keep going. You're crushing it—even if "crushing it" sometimes involves crushing a bag of chips. Balance, right?

9.54. Take Breaks as Needed

Taking breaks during your weight management journey isn't just okay—it's mandatory. Your body isn't a machine, and even machines overheat. If you're feeling burned out, exhausted, or like you might spontaneously combust at the sight of a treadmill, congratulations—you're human. It's time to hit pause.

But let me be clear: a break isn't a failure. It's like a pit stop in a race—you're just refuelling, not quitting. Use the time to rediscover what it's like to exist without gym clothes and protein bars. Read a book, binge a questionable TV show, meditate, or have a meaningful conversation with your couch. Bonus points if you can do all of the above without accidentally scrolling through #FitnessInfluencer on Instagram.

Self-care isn't a weakness. It's an Olympic-level skill. Balancing ambition with recovery is how you stay in the game long-term. So, if your body says, *"Hey, maybe we don't deadlift our emotional baggage today,"* listen to it.

When you're ready to return, you'll do so with a vengeance (and possibly a newfound appreciation for sweatpants). Rested, recharged, and ready to crush it again. Because remember: even superheroes take a break—they just don't post it on Instagram.

10. Last Word

As we stumble to the finish line of this weight-management magnum opus, let's take a moment to reflect on what a wild ride it's been. Who knew the secret to lasting change wasn't choking down celery sticks or trying to sweat your soul out on a treadmill at 5 a.m.? No, my friend, it's about balance—a mythical unicorn of a concept that somehow involves eating vegetables and not losing your mind.

These pages haven't just been a guide; they've been a reality check. This book has shown you the long game, from decoding the hormonal circus in your body to tearing apart new diets with the precision of a frustrated chef hacking at a raw spaghetti squash. Spoiler alert: quick fixes lie to you, just like your ex, who said they'd change.

Let's face it—life is chaos, and you're trying to balance it all like a clown juggling flaming swords while riding a unicycle. Some days, you'll be that clown; others, you'll be the flaming sword. It's fine. The point is to keep showing up, even if you're just rolling in with half a salad and a vague plan to do yoga while binge-watching Orange is the New Black.

This isn't a one-size-fits-all solution because you're not a one-size-fits-all person. You're a wonderfully complicated, slightly messy human with unique quirks, challenges, and a penchant for midnight snacks you swore you wouldn't eat. Own it. Your journey is yours, even if it sometimes feels like a bad reality show with too many plot twists.

As you wrap this up, remember that balance isn't about perfection. It's about not falling flat on your face every time life trips you up. Sometimes, you'll eat kale; other times, you'll eat cake. The key is not letting one slice of cake spiral into a week of unhinged decisions. Progress, not perfection, my friend.

So, here's to your journey—your perfectly imperfect, gloriously flawed, and hilariously unique journey. May you find joy in your successes, laugh at your failures, and keep moving forward, even if it's with a slice of pizza in hand and a slightly smug grin because you're still crushing it. Cheers to you, the chaotic, determined, and fabulous human you are. You've got this. Or not. Either way, it's okay.

THE END

www.ingramcontent.com/pod-product-compliance
Lightning Source LLC
Chambersburg PA
CBHW071217210326
41597CB00016B/1843